3D Shape

3D Shape

Its Unique Place in Visual Perception

Zygmunt Pizlo

The MIT Press
Cambridge, Massachusetts
London, England

For information about special quantity discounts, please email special_sales@ mitpress.mit.edu.

This book was set in Stone Sans and Stone Serif by SNP Best-set Typesetter Ltd., Hong Kong.
Printed and bound in the United States of America.

Library of Congress Cataloging-in-Publication Data

Pizlo, Zygmunt.
3D shape : its unique place in visual perception / Zygmunt Pizlo.
    p.   cm.
Includes bibliographical references and index.
ISBN 978-0-262-16251-7 (hardcover : alk. paper)
1. Form perception. 2. Visual perception. I. Title.
BF293.P59 2008
152.14′23—dc22

                                                                  2007039869

10 9 8 7 6 5 4 3 2 1

This book is dedicated to Prof. Robert M. Steinman, teacher, collaborator, and friend, whose questions and suggestions made this book possible.

Contents

4 Formalisms Enter into the Study of Shape Perception   115

5 A New Paradigm for Studying Shape Perception   145

Preface

This book is the very first devoted exclusively to the perception of shape by human beings and machines. This claim will surely be surprising to many, perhaps most, readers, but it is true nonetheless. Why is this the first such book? I know of only one good reason. Namely, the fact that shape is a unique perceptual property was not appreciated, and until it was, it was not apparent that shape should be treated separately from all other perceptual properties, such as depth, motion, speed, and color. Shape is special because it is both complex and structured. These two characteristics are responsible for the fact that shapes are perceived veridically, that is, perceived as they really are "out there." The failure to appreciate the unique status of shape in visual perception led to methodological errors when attempts were made to study shape, arguably the most important perceptual property of many objects. These errors resulted in a large conflicting literature that made it impossible to develop a coherent theoretical treatment of this unique perceptual property. Even a good working definition of shape was wanting. What got me interested in trying to understand this unique, but poorly defined, property of objects?

My interest began when I was working on an engineering application, a doctoral project in electrical engineering that involved formulating statistical methods for pattern recognition. Pattern recognition was known to be an important tool for detecting anomalies in the manufacture of integrated circuits. The task of an engineer on a production line is like the task of a medical doctor; both have to diagnose the presence and the nature of a problem based on the pattern of data provided by "signs." I realized shortly after beginning to work on this problem that it was very difficult to write a pattern recognition algorithm "smart" enough to accomplish what an engineer did very easily just by looking at histograms and scatter plots. It became obvious to me that before one could make computers discriminate one pattern from another, one might have to understand how humans manage to do this so well. This epiphany came over me on the night before I defended my first doctoral dissertation. My interest in studying human shape perception started during the early morning hours of that memorable day as I tried to anticipate issues likely to come up at my defense.

Studying pattern and shape perception requires more than a cursory knowledge of geometry, both Euclidean and projective. It also requires the ability to apply this knowledge to a perspective projection from a three-dimensional (3D) space to a two-dimensional (2D) image. I had a reasonable background in electrical engineering, but it did not include projective geometry. I had to learn it from scratch. It took both time and effort, but it paid off. At the time I did not realize that this was unusual. It never occurred to me that anyone would try to study shape, the topic that served for my second doctoral degree, without knowing geometry quite well.

My formal study of human shape perception was done in the Sensori-Neural and Perceptual Processes Program (SNAPP) of the Psychology Department at the University of Maryland at College Park where Robert M. Steinman served as my doctoral advisor. My dissertation also benefited a great deal from interactions with several members of the Center for Automation Research and Computer Science at this institution. My independent study of projective geometry was greatly facilitated by numerous discussions with Isaac Weiss. Realize that I was starting from scratch. I was analyzing known properties of geometrical optics simultaneously with learning about groups, transformations, and invariants. Here, my limited formal background in geometry led me to stumble onto some new aspects of projective geometry that had not been explored before. I was encouraged to pursue this path by Azriel Rosenfeld, my second doctoral mentor, who was affiliated with SNAPP. Azriel Rosenfeld, who was well-known for his many contributions to machine vision, was a mathematician by training. He was always interested in exploring the limits of mathematical knowledge and of mathematical formalisms, and he, Isaac Weiss, and I published some of our insights about a new type of perspective invariants that grew out of my dissertation. After mastering what I needed to understand in projective geometry, and after developing the new geometrical tools needed for a model of the perspective projection in the human eye,

I realized that I should also learn regularization theory with elements of the calculus of variations. Learning this part of mathematics was facilitated by interactions with Yannis Aloimonos, who was among the first to apply this formalism in computer vision. He asked me, now almost 20 years ago, whether regularization theory is the right formalism for understanding human vision. I answered then that I was not sure. My answer now is "Yes" for reasons made abundantly clear in this book. My interactions and learning experiences during my graduate education at the University of Maryland at College Park were not limited to geometry and regularization theory. From Azriel Rosenfeld I learned about pyramid models of figure–ground organization, and I learned about computational applications of Biederman's and Pentland's theories of shape from Sven Dickinson. Both figure prominently in my treatment of shape presented in this book. Now that the reader knows the circuitous route that led me to study human shape perception, I will explain why I decided to write this book.

The primary motivation for writing it grew out of my teaching obligations. When I began to teach, I tried to present the topic called "shape perception" as if it were a traditional topic within the specialty called "perception." As such, shape perception, like other topics such as color perception, should be taught on the basis of the accumulation of specialized knowledge. Clearly, the history of a topic in a scientific specialty, such as shape perception, should be more than a collection of names, theories, and experimental results. The history of the topic should reveal progress in our understanding of the relevant phenomena. I found it impossible to demonstrate the accumulation of knowledge in the area called "shape perception." The existing literature did not allow a coherent story, and I decided to try to figure out what was going on. Knowing this was important for doing productive research, as well as for teaching. How do you decide to take the *next step* toward understanding shape when where the last step left you was unclear? Recognizing that shape is a special perceptual property did the trick. It made both teaching and productive research possible. This book describes how much we currently understand about shape and how we came to reach the point that we have reached. It is a long story with many twists and turns. I found it an exciting adventure and hope that the reader experiences it this way, too.

By trying to maintain the focus of my presentation, I deliberately left out material that ordinarily would have been included if I were writing a comprehensive review of visual perception, rather than a book on the specialized topic called "shape perception." Specifically, I did not include a treatment of the neuroanatomy or neurophysiology of shape perception. Little is known about shape at this level of analysis because we are only now in a position to begin to ask appropriate questions. The emphasis of the book is on understanding perceptual mechanisms, rather than on brain localization. For example, the currently available knowledge of neurophysiology cannot inform us about which "cost function" is being minimized when a 3D shape percept is produced. I also did not include a large body of evidence on the perception of 2D patterns and 3D scenes that is only tangentially relevant to our understanding of the perception of 3D shapes.

The text concentrates on the discussion of the main concepts; technical material has been reduced to a minimum. This made it possible to tell the "story of shape" without interruption. A full understanding of the material contained in this book, however, requires understanding the underlying technical details. The appendices provide the basic mathematical and computational information that should be sufficient for the reader to achieve a technical understanding of the infrastructure that provided the basis for my treatment of shape. The references to sources contained in these appendices can also serve as a starting point for more in-depth readings in geometry and computational vision, readings that I hope will encourage individuals to undertake additional work on this unique perceptual property. Much remains to be done.

I had six goals when I began writing this book, namely, I set out to (i) critically review *all* prior research on shape; (ii) remove apparent contradictions among experimental results; (iii) compare several theories, computational and noncomputational, to each other, as well as to dozens of psychophysical results; (iv) present a new theory of shape; (v) show that this new theory is consistent with all prior and new results on shape perception; and (vi) set the stage for *meaningful* future research on shape. My choice of these particular goals and the degree to which I have been successful in reaching each of them can only be evaluated by reading the book. Obviously, my success with each goal is less important than my success in (i) encouraging the reader to think deeply about the nature and significance of shape perception and (ii) stimulating productive research on this fundamental perceptual problem.

The new theory presented in this book shows how a 3D shape percept is produced from a 2D retinal image, assuming only that the image has been *organized* into 2D shapes. One can argue that this new theory is able to solve the most difficult aspect of 3D shape perception. What remains to be done is to explain how the 2D shapes on the retina are *organized*. The process that accomplishes this, called "figure–ground organization" by the Gestalt psychologists, is not dealt with in great detail in this book, simply because not much is known about it at this writing. It is likely, however, that now that I have called attention to the importance of this critical organizing process in shape perception, it will be easier to (i) expand our understanding of how it works and (ii) formulate plausible computational models of the mechanisms that allow human beings to perceive the shapes of objects veridically.

I will conclude this preface by acknowledging individuals who contributed to this book and to the research that made it possible, beginning with the contributions of my students: Monika Salach-Golyska, Michael Scheessele, Moses Chan, Adam Stevenson, and Kirk Loubier worked with me on shape perception and figure–ground organization; Yunfeng Li designed and conducted recent psychophysical experiments on a number of aspects of shape and helped me formulate and test the current computational model; and he, along with Emil Stefanov and Jack Saalweachter, helped prepare the graphical material used in this book.

I also acknowledge the contributions of the late Julie Epelboim, who was a valuable colleague at the University of Maryland, where she served as a subject in my work on pyramid models and perspective invariants. My son, Filip Pizlo, contributed to a number of aspects of my shape research. He helped write programs for our psychophysical experiments and was instrumental in designing demos illustrating many of the key concepts. Interactions with my colleagues, Charles Bouman, Edward Delp, Sven Dickinson, Gregory Francis, Christoph Hoffmann, Walter Kropatsch, Longin Jan Latecki, Robert Nowack, Voicu Popescu, and Karthik Ramani contributed to my understanding of inverse problems, regularization theory, shape perception, geometrical modeling, and figure–ground organization. I also acknowledge the suggestion and encouragement to write a book like this that I received from George Sperling and Misha Pavel after a talk on the history of shape research that I gave at the 25th Annual Interdisciplinary Conference at Jackson Hole in 2000. None of these individuals are responsible for any imperfections, errors, or omissions present in this book.

I acknowledge support from the National Science Foundation, National Institutes of Health, the Air Force Office of Scientific Research, and the Department of Energy for my research and for writing this book. I thank Barbara Murphy, Kate Blakinger, Meagan Stacey, and Katherine Almeida at MIT Press for editorial assistance.

Finally, I thank my family for their understanding and support while my mind was bent out of shape by concentrating excessively on this unique perceptual property.

3D Shape

1 Early Theories of Shape and the First Experiments on Shape Constancy

1.1 Shape Is Special

This book is concerned with the perception of shape. "Perception" can be defined simply—namely, as becoming aware of the external world through the action of the senses. "Shape," unlike perception, cannot be defined in such simple terms, and much of this book is devoted to explaining why this is the case, how it came to pass, and how we have finally reached a point where we can discuss and study shape in a way that captures the significance of this critical property of objects. When we refer to the "shape" of an object, we mean those geometrical characteristics of a specific three-dimensional (3D) object that make it possible to perceive the object veridically from many different viewing directions, that is, to perceive it as it actually is in the world "out there." Understanding how the human visual system accomplishes this is essential for understanding the mechanisms underlying shape perception. Understanding this is also essential if we want to build machines that can see shapes as humans do.

Understanding shape perception is of fundamental importance. Why? Shape *is* fundamental because it provides human beings with accurate information about objects "out there." Accurate information about the nature of objects "out there" is essential for effective interactions with them. An object's shape is a *unique* perceptual property of the object in the sense that it is the *only* perceptual property that has sufficient complexity to allow an object to be identified. Furthermore, shape's high degree of complexity makes it quite different from *all* other perceptual properties. For example, color varies along only three dimensions: hue, brightness, and saturation. Many objects "out there" will have the same color. Other perceptual properties are even simpler: An object's size and weight can vary only along a single dimension, and many objects will have the same size or weight. Shape is unlike all of these properties because it is much more complex. An object's shape can be described along a large number of dimensions. Imagine how many points on the contour of a circle would have to be moved to transform the circle into the outline of a human silhouette or how many points on the outline of the silhouette would have to be moved to change its outline into a circle. When two shapes are very different, as they are in figure 1.1, the position of almost all points along their contours would have to be changed to change the shape of one to the shape of the other. The circle and the inscribed silhouette of a human being are about as different as any two shapes can be. All of the points except those where the human silhouette touches the circle (the tips of the fingers and the soles of the feet) would have to be moved to change one to the other. Theoretically, the number of points along an outline is infinite, so the number of dimensions characterizing an arbitrary shape is, theoretically, infinitely large. Fortunately, in the world of living things like ourselves, one need not deal with an infinite number of dimensions because

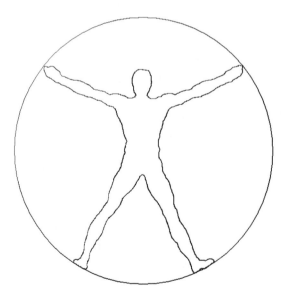

Figure 1.1
A human silhouette and a circumscribed circle (after Leonardo DaVinci).

the human being's sensory systems are constrained. Even in the fovea, where the highest density of cells in the retina is found, there are only about 400 receptor cells per millimeter (Polyak, 1957). Thus, when a circular shape with a diameter of 1 deg of visual angle is projected on the fovea, only 300 or 400 receptors would receive information about the circle's contour. It is clear, however, that despite such constraints, sufficient information would remain to disambiguate all objects human beings have encountered within the environment in which they evolved and are likely to encounter in the future. Once this is appreciated, it becomes clear that what we call "shape" has considerable evolutionary significance because the function of very many objects is conveyed primarily by their shape.

Naturally occurring objects tend to fall into similarly shaped groups, and this makes it convenient to deal with them as members of families of similar shapes. Most apples look alike, and most cars look alike. Note that when you view your car from a new angle, its image on your retina changes, but it is perceived as the same car. This fact defines what is called "shape constancy." Formally, "shape constancy" refers to the fact that the percept of the shape of a given object remains constant despite changes in the shape of the object's retinal image. The shape of the retinal image changes when the viewing orientation changes.[1] Shape constancy is a fundamental perceptual phenomenon, and much of this book is devoted to explaining conditions under which shape constancy can be reliably achieved and the mechanisms underlying this accomplishment. Shape constancy has profound significance because the perceived shape of a given object is veridical (the way it is "out there") despite the fact that its shape on the retina, the plane in which it stimulates our visual receptors, has changed. These considerations apply to many shape families. Figure 1.2 shows two views of the same scene, each taken from a different viewpoint. It is easy to recognize all of the individual objects in each view. Determining which contours and which regions of an image correspond to a single object is called "figure–ground organization." This terminology and its role in shape constancy was introduced by the Gestalt psychologists. It will be discussed later when their contributions are described. Interestingly, both figure–ground organization and shape constancy can be achieved when only the contours of objects are visible, as can be seen in figure 1.3. Surface details and structure are not needed to recognize a

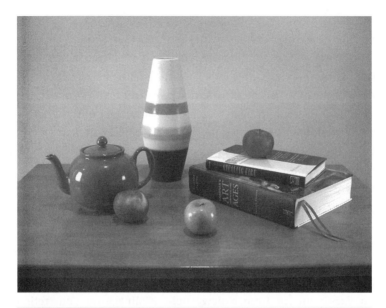

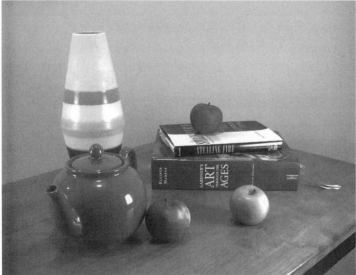

Figure 1.2
Two views of an indoor scene illustrating two fundamental perceptual phenomena.
"Figure–ground organization" is illustrated by the fact that it is easy to determine
which regions and contours in the image correspond to individual objects. Note,
also, that the contour in the image belongs to the region representing the object.
"Shape constancy" is illustrated by the fact that it is easy to recognize the shapes of
objects regardless of the viewing direction (photo by D. Black).

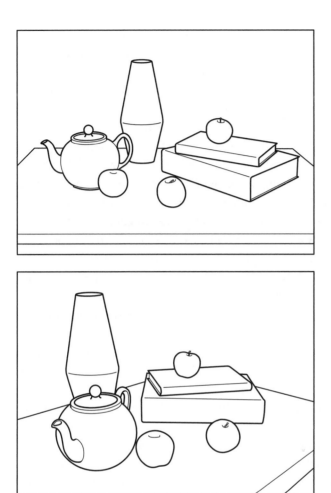

Figure 1.3
Line drawing version of the previous figure (prepared by D. Black).

variety of individual objects. Retinal shape, alone, is sufficient for shape recognition and shape constancy.

Note, however, that two shape families, ellipses and triangles, are quite different, and, as you will see, failure to appreciate this difference can make a lot of trouble. Ellipses and triangles are very much simpler than all other shapes. They do not offer the degree of complexity required by the visual system to achieve shape constancy. A shape selected from the family of ellipses requires only one parameter, its aspect ratio (the ratio of the lengths of the long and short axis), for a unique identification of a particular ellipse. Changing the magnitude of the two axes, while keeping their ratio constant, changes only the size of an ellipse, not its shape. The family of triangular shapes requires only two parameters (triangular shape is uniquely specified by two angles because the three angles in a triangle always sum to 180 deg). Note that the number of parameters needed to describe shape within these two families (ellipses and triangles) is small, similar in number to the parameters required to describe color, size, and weight. Much was made above about how a high degree of complexity makes shape special in that it can provide a basis for the accurate identification of objects. Clearly, using ellipses and triangles to study shape might present a problem because their shapes are characterized by only one or two parameters. It has. It held the field back for more than half a century (1931–1991).

Why do ellipses and triangles present problems? They present problems because the 3D world is represented in only two dimensions on the retina. The Bishop Berkeley (1709) emphasized that a perspective transformation from the world to the retina reduces the amount of information available for the identification of both objects and depth. Note that this loss affects ellipses and triangles profoundly. Any ellipse "out there" will, at various orientations, be able to produce any ellipse on the retina. This fact is illustrated in figure 1.4a. Here two ellipses with different shapes are shown at the top, and their retinal images are shown at the bottom. The retinal images have identical shapes because the taller ellipse was slanted more. Similarly, any triangle "out there" can produce any triangle on the retina. Note that these are the *only* two families of shapes that confound the shape itself with the viewing orientation. They do this because a perspective transformation from 3D to two dimensions (2D) changes the shape of a 2D (flat or planar) shape with only two degrees of freedom (see appendix A, section A.1). It follows that if the shape itself is characterized by only one or two parameters (as ellipses and triangles are), the information about their shape is completely lost during their projection to the retina and shape constancy may become difficult, even impossible, to achieve. However, if the shape of a figure is characterized by more than two parameters, perspective projection does not eliminate all of the shape information, and shape constancy can almost always be achieved. This is true for any family of shapes, other than ellipses and triangles. The simplest family in which constancy can be achieved reliably is the family of rectangles. In

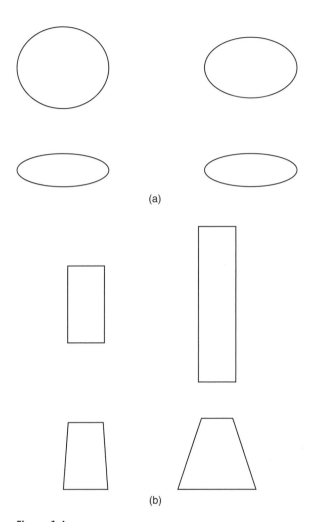

(a)

(b)

Figure 1.4
(a) Ellipses with different shapes (top) can produce identical retinal images (bottom). The ellipse on the top left was slanted around the horizontal axis more than the ellipse on the top right. As a result, their retinal images (bottom) are identical. (b) Rectangles with different shapes cannot produce identical retinal images. The rectangle on the top right was slanted around the horizontal axis more than the rectangle on the top left. As a result, the heights of their retinal images (bottom) are identical, but their shapes are not. Specifically, the angles in the two retinal images are different. If the slant of the rectangle on the top right were equal to that of the rectangle on the top left, the angles in the retinal images would be identical, but the heights would be different. This means that the shapes of the retinal images would be different, as well.

figure 1.4b, two rectangles with different shapes are shown at the top, and their retinal images are shown at the bottom. The taller rectangle had to be slanted more than the shorter one, to produce images with the same heights, but despite the fact that the heights of the retinal images are the same, the angles are not. In fact, two rectangles with different shapes can *never* produce identical retinal images. More generally, if two figures or objects have different shapes, they are very unlikely to produce identical retinal images, as long as the figures are not ellipses or triangles. It follows that understanding shape constancy cannot be based on experiments in which ellipses or triangles were used. This fact, which was overlooked until very recently, has led to a lot of confusion in the literature on shape perception. Note that this confusion might have been avoided because a formal treatment of the rules for making perspective projections (rules that reveal the confound of shape and viewing orientation) had been used by artists since the beginning of the fifteenth century (see Kemp, 1990), and the mathematics of projective geometry had been worked out quite completely by the end of the nineteenth century (Klein, 1939). Why was this confound ignored until recently by those who studied shape perception? The answer lies in the fact that the people who made this mistake did not come to their studies of shape from art or mathematics. They came from a quite different tradition, a tradition that will be described next.

1.2   Explaining Visual Constancies with a "Taking into Account" Principle

Formal research on shape did not start until the beginning of the twentieth century, after the Gestalt Revolution had been launched. By that time, the perception of other important properties of objects such as color, size, lightness, and motion had been studied intensively and very successfully for almost 100 years. For each of these properties a perceptual "constancy" had been defined: The percept of a surface's lightness and color, of an object's size, and of its speed, had been shown to remain approximately constant despite changes in its retinal image. These changes of the retinal image could be brought about by changes in the spectrum and intensity of the illuminating light, and by changes of the viewing distance. The conceptual framework and research questions adopted for the study of shape constancy were based on these successful studies of other perceptual constancies. However, generalizing existing knowledge and borrowing an experimental methodology from simple perceptual properties such as color and size to shape, which is a complex multidimensional property, was unwarranted, and dangerous as well. Could this mistake have been avoided? Perhaps. When the formal study of shape started with Thouless' (1931a, b) experiments, existing experimental results had already suggested that the mechanisms underlying shape perception were likely to be different from those underlying size, speed, and lightness, but many students of shape perception mistakenly assumed that shape is like all other visual properties. This *encouraged* them to try to confirm, rather than to question, their theory of shape constancy, which made use of other perceptual properties, when they began to do experiments on shape perception. Their commitment to this assumption caused them to ignore some important aspects of their results. Assuming that shape was like other perceptual properties prevented them from appreciating what was actually going on in their experiments. Had they considered the possibility that shape is fundamentally different from the simpler perceptual properties, they probably would have noticed important, unusual patterns in their data.

The conceptual framework for Thouless' (1931a, b) study of shape can be traced back a long way. His approach was derived from philosophical discussions of epistemological problems reaching back to Alhazen (1083) in the eleventh century. Highlights of these discussions will be presented here because they will allow the reader to appreciate why Thouless and many other modern researchers adopted the particular type of explanation of the perceptual constancies they did. They adopted "taking into account" explanations of lightness, color, and size and expected to be able to extend this approach to their studies of shape constancy as well. Traditionally, all of these perceptual constancies were explained by "taking into account" contextual information present in the viewing conditions. For example, size constancy was "explained" by taking viewing distance into account. Lightness constancy was explained by taking cues to illumination into account, and so forth. Contextual information was critical because the retinal image was *ambiguous*.

The recorded history of the perceptual constancies began long ago with Alhazen (1083), whose book was the first work known to the author to raise the problem of shape constancy. Alhazen, who lived in the second half of the tenth and the first half of the eleventh centuries, is generally viewed as representing a bridge between the science of the ancient Greek philosophers and the precursors of modern science following the European Renaissance. Alhazen made many fundamental contributions to the study of vision. Unfortunately, most were either overlooked during the development of modern science in Europe, which took place between the seventeenth and twentieth centuries, or are not mentioned in contemporary reviews of the history of the subject (Sabra, 1989, 1994; Howard, 1996). To illustrate, Alhazen performed the first systematic observations of afterimages (Alhazen, 1083, p. 51). He also reported the dependence of visual acuity on luminance (p. 54). In addition, he described mixing colors (pp. 144–5) with a precursor of Maxwell's top. He also described color constancy (pp. 141–2), shape constancy (p. 279), and position constancy (pp. 193–4). He conjectured that what came to be called "unconscious inference" in the nineteenth century explained all of these important perceptual phenomena (p. 136). He also discussed the perceived size/perceived distance relationship and its role in size constancy (p. 177). Alhazen even described what we now call "Panum's fusional area" in his discussion of binocular vision (p. 240).[2] Alhazen did not perform systematic experiments to verify his claims, but he described many important perceptual phenomena and recognized the operation of several perceptual mechanisms. Most subsequent writers seldom credited his contributions.

In Europe, the thirteenth century marks the revival of philosophy and the beginnings of what came to be called "science" in Europe. This revival was facilitated by the founding of the first European universities in Bologna, Paris, and Oxford in eleventh and twelfth centuries and a number of others soon after. Philosophers and mathematicians, such as Grosseteste, Bacon, and Peckham in England, Witelo in Poland, and Aquinas and Bonaventure in Italy, stimulated interest in natural sciences by translating old works from Arabic into Latin, as well as contributing new ideas (Hamlyn, 1961; Howard & Rogers, 1995). However, modern philosophy and the scientific study of perception did not start until the seventeenth century when Descartes (1596–1650) came on the scene. Descartes contributed to several areas of knowledge. In philosophy, he offered a dualistic, interactionist interpretation of the mind–body problem and a nativistic view of the origin of our knowledge about the external world (time, space, and motion). In mathematics, he founded analytic geometry. In physiology, he introduced the concept of reflex action and distinguished what came to be called "sensory and motor mechanisms" in the nervous system. Only his contributions to the psychology of visual perception will be discussed here.

Descartes distinguished the mental faculties called "perception" (becoming aware), "cognition" (knowing and understanding), and "conation" (willing). The shapes of objects are, according to Descartes, perceived intuitively in an essentially passive act. The rules of geometrical optics are also intuited. Descartes (1637) published his views on spatial vision in Discourse on Method, Optics, Geometry, and Meteorology. In this book, Descartes discussed the problem presented by the inversion of the retinal image produced by the eyes' lens, cues to depth, and size and shape constancy. For these constancies he, like Alhazen, offered a "taking into account" explanation, the explanation that will dominate virtually all thinking about perceptual constancies in the nineteenth and twentieth centuries. His treatment of "taking into account" goes as follows: It begins with a discussion of Kepler's (1604) book *Comments on Witelo*, in which the rules of image formation predicted that the retinal image was inverted. Kepler's prediction was verified empirically by Scheiner in 1625 and by Descartes in 1637. It raises a problem, namely, we perceive an object as "right side up" despite the fact that its retinal image is "upside down." Descartes analyzed this problem by using an analogy from tactual perception. When a blind man holds a stick in each hand, and when he knows that the sticks form an X, the man not only has knowledge of the positions of his hands but he also can infer knowledge of the positions of the ends of the sticks. Once he knows that the sticks are crossed, he knows that the tip of the stick on the right is on the left side of his body and that the tip of the stick on the left is on the right side (see figure 1.5). According to Descartes, having such knowledge (the rules of geometry) a priori is critical for solving this problem. It allows the blind man to draw the correct inference about the spatial position of the ends of the sticks. Thus, for example, while keeping the two sticks crossed, if he touches an object with a stick that he holds in his right hand, he would naturally know that the object is on the left. Here, the perception of left and right in physical space is not determined by the positions of the left and right parts of the body (hands in this example). Thus, it was not surprising to Descartes that the mind perceives up versus down, as well as right versus left, in the physical world correctly, despite the fact that the retinal image is inverted. This visual example is clearly analogous to the example of the blind man holding

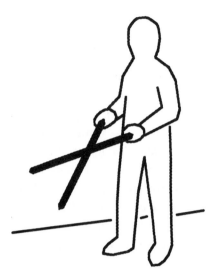

Figure 1.5
A blind man using sticks can correctly judge left and right "out there" despite the fact that left "out there" is actually sensed by his right hand (after Descartes, 1637).

sticks because the visual rays intersect within the eye before they hit the retina. However, note that Descartes adopted a view that perception of the location of an object "out there" involves inferences or thinking. The question remains how the visual system knows that the visual rays intersect before they hit the retina without reading Kepler's book. For Descartes, this did not present a problem because he considered such knowledge to be innate.

Descartes went on to describe ocular vergence as a cue to distance. Again, he used an analogy of a blind man who, with two sticks, can judge the distance of an object by triangulation. The man does this by means of a "natural geometry" made possible by the fact that he knows the distance between his hands and the angles each stick makes with the line connecting his hands. In the case of visual triangulation, the distance between the hands is analogous to the distance between the two eyes, and the angles between the sticks are analogous to the angles formed by the line of sight of each eye with the line connecting the two eyes. Specifically, the length of one side in a triangle, together with sizes of two angles, allow solving the triangle, including the computation of its height, which in this case corresponds to the viewing distance. Descartes goes on to give another example of how the blind man, who represents the visual system, can solve the triangulation problem in the case of motion parallax, that is, when an observer moves relative to some object. Note that in both cases, Descartes, like Alhazen, proposed that these problems were solved by *unconscious* thought processes.

Locke (1690), along with Hobbes (1651), is credited with founding British empiricism. Locke formulated an alternative view of perception, namely, he, in contrast to Descartes, conjectured that all knowledge is derived from experience. He completely rejected Descartes' assumption of innate ideas. He held that a human being's mind begins as a "tabula rasa" (a blank page), and experience with recurring sensations leads to the learning of simple ideas, which are then elaborated into complex ideas by additional associations. For Locke, perceptions of such basic things as shape and motion were complex ideas. Locke claimed that the rules of association, described by Aristotle, provide the mechanisms underlying perception. For Locke, unlike Descartes, perceptual constancies have to be learned.

Molyneux (1692), a friend of Locke, shared his rejection of innate ideas. He supported this claim by posing the following problem. Assume that a person born blind learned to identify and discriminate among objects by the sense of touch. In particular, assume that the person can correctly identify a sphere and a cube. Now suppose that the blind person is made to see. Will the person be able to tell which object is a sphere and which is a cube using vision alone, without touching the objects? Molyneux claimed that the person will not be able to identify these objects. The reason, according to Molyneux, is that the blind person did not have a chance to learn how to see. Molyneux's thought experiment was to receive a lot of attention in 1960s when von Senden's (1932/1960) book on the vision of newly sighted patients came under critical review (Zuckerman & Rock, 1957).

Berkeley, in his *A New Theory of Vision*, published in 1709, elaborated Locke's and Molyneux's empiricism. For Berkeley, vision was always uncertain because it, like hearing, sensed things at a distance. The shapes and sizes of objects had to be learned by comparing visual sensations to touch sensations, which provided a direct and, therefore, reliable source of information. *Only* tactual perception, along with the sensations from the muscles that moved the hands during tactual exploration, can provide direct information about the environment. He illustrates this by pointing out that the perspective projection from the 3D environment to the 2D retina does not preserve information about depth: A point on the retina could be an image of any of the infinitely many points along the line emanating from the point on the retina and proceeding to the object. A newborn human being has no way of judging distances given visually. In essence, according to Berkeley, the visual perception of distance is learned by forming sensorimotor associations. Specifically, when an observer looks at an object binocularly, the line of sight of each eye is directed toward the object, forming an angle called "vergence." The observer is aware of the angle by feeling the state of his eye muscles, and when the observer walks toward the object, the angle changes and the sensations associated with change are noticed. The relation between the sensations from the eye muscles and the number of steps required to reach the object is learned, stored, and used later by means of what we would call today a "look-up table" to provide the mechanism underlying the perception of distance. Similarly, haptics (movements, positions, and orientations of the hands) associated with manipulating objects can provide a basis for creating look-up tables for the shapes of different objects and for the orientation of surfaces. In other words, the individual need not solve geometrical problems to "take into account" environmental characteristics once appropriate look-up tables have been established by associative learning. Berkeley's suggestion has become the standard way of formulating "taking into account" explanations by empiricists ever since his day.

1.3 Helmholtz' Influence When the Modern Era Began

The next important development appeared about 150 years later when Helmholtz published his *Treatise on Physiological Optics* (1867/2000), in which he takes on these problems at what is generally accepted as the beginning of the modern scientific era: He addressed the question of how sensations produced by stimulation of the retina lead to perceptions of 3D space. Helmholtz' approach, like Berkeley's, was empiristic. He supported his teacher's, Johannes Müller's, claims about case histories of persons who were born blind and whose vision was restored by surgery (Helmholtz, 1867/2000, volume 3, pp. 220–7). Such persons, who did not have any prior visual experience, were said to be unable to discriminate among shapes and spatial relations. Helmholtz confirmed these claims and concluded that these patients, like newborn babies, had to learn how to see. He suggested that learning how to see was accomplished by making repetitive eye movements along contours of shapes, an idea that was to be used almost a century later by Hebb (1949).

How did Helmholtz apply his empiristic views to the perceptual constancies? According to Helmholtz, visual perception is derived from "unconscious conclusions" about the external world. These conclusions are reached by means of associations of sensations and memory traces. For example, we come to learn to appreciate the locations of objects in space in the following way:

When those nervous mechanisms whose terminals lie on the right-hand portions of the retinas of the two eyes have been stimulated, our usual experience, repeated a million times all through life, has been that a luminous object was over there in front of us on our left. We had to lift the hand toward the left to hide the light or to grasp the luminous object; or we had to move toward the left to get closer to it. Thus while in these cases no particular conscious conclusion may be present, yet the essential and original office of such a conclusion has been performed, and the result of it has been attained; simply, of course, by the unconscious process of association of ideas going on in the dark background of our memory. (Helmholtz, 1867/2000, volume 3, p. 26, translated by Southall)

The concept of "unconscious conclusion" is perhaps *the* critical concept in Helmholtz' theory of perception.[3] Binocular depth perception can provide another example of how it was used by Helmholtz. Namely, each point in the environment produces a retinal image in the observer's left and right eye. Assume that the observer's visual system knows accurately and precisely the orientation and position of one eye relative to the other. In such a case, the 3D position of the physical point can be computed as an intersection of the visual rays emanating from the retinal points (volume 3, p. 155). This should remind the reader of Descartes' explanation described above. The difference between Helmholtz' and Descartes' formulation was that Helmholtz does not subscribe to Descartes' notion that the human being has an innate understanding of geometry. Instead, he adopts Berkeley's approach in which a look-up table is established between sensations and their significance "out there."

Now, let us examine Helmholtz' views on shape perception. They are probably best expressed in the following paragraph from his "Review of the Theories" section of his *Treatise*:

an idea of an individual object . . . includes all the possible single aggregates of sensation which can be produced by this object when we view it on different sides and
touch it or examine it in other ways. This is the actual, the real content of any such
idea of a definite object. It has no other; and on the assumption of the data above
mentioned, this content can undoubtedly be obtained by experience. The only
psychic activity required for this purpose is the regularly recurrent association
between two ideas which have often been connected before. The oftener this association recurs, the more firm and obligatory it becomes. (volume 3, pp. 533–4).

Thus, according to Helmholtz, the memory of a 3D shape (its mental
representation) involves a collection of 2D images of the shape (plus
tactual sensations) obtained from different viewing directions. Subsequent
recognition of the shape involves matching the current view with the
stored views (volume 3, p. 23). There is very little additional discussion of
shape perception in Helmholtz' three-volume *Treatise*, at most a paragraph
or two.

Now that we have an idea of the prevailing views when the modern
study of shape perception began, we can turn to a discussion of the first
experimental study of shape perception. It was performed in a period in
which Helmholtz' ideas were taken very seriously.

1.4   Thouless' Misleading Experiments

Thouless' two papers, published in 1931, were the most influential, albeit
misleading, contributions in the history of shape constancy (Thouless,
1931a, b). These papers are cited in all textbooks of perception known to
the author. The significance of these papers stems from the fact that Thouless concluded, and was widely believed to have demonstrated, that shape
constancy involves "taking slant into account" ("slant" is defined as the
angle between the frontal plane and the plane containing the test figure).
He actually did not do this. This claim requires a detailed description
of Thouless' papers. Once this is done, Thouless' "contribution" will be
evaluated.

In his first experiment, Thouless used two figures, a circle and a square,
and tested the accuracy of shape perception of each figure when the figure
was presented at a slant (Thouless, 1931a). One *should* expect different
outcomes with these two shapes. Remember that the family of ellipses to
which the circle belongs (a circle is an ellipse with aspect ratio of one),
is completely characterized by only *one* parameter. You must also keep in

mind that the family of perspective projections changes the shape of a figure with two degrees of freedom. It follows that in the case of ellipses (one of the two stimuli used by Thouless), the retinal image completely confounds the shape of the figure with its viewing orientation. That is, *any* ellipse "out there" can produce *any* ellipse on the retina (figure 1.4a). Squares, which are in the family of "quadrilaterals," are very different. They are characterized by *four* parameters (ratio of lengths of two sides, plus three angles). As a result, even though the retinal image of a rectangle is affected by slant, its image does not confound the shape of a rectangle with its slant (figure 1.4b). Clearly, ellipses and rectangles should lead to very different results in a shape constancy experiment.

The test figure (a square or a circle) was put on a table. The subject viewed the figure binocularly and was asked to draw its shape. If the percept of the slanted figure were veridical, the reproduced and the presented shapes would have been identical. In particular, their aspect ratios would be the same. The aspect ratios produced were greater than the retinal aspect ratio, but lower than the physical aspect ratio. Thus, perfect shape constancy was not obtained with either figure, but shape constancy was less accurate (larger systematic error) and less reliable (more variable across trials) with the circle than with the square. The fact that shape constancy was not perfect was to be expected—similar results had already been obtained in size, lightness, and color constancy experiments. What was not expected was the difference in the amount of constancy between the circle and the square. This result cannot be easily explained by the "taking slant into account" theory because in this theory, the perceived slant and, hence, the degree of shape constancy do not depend on the shape itself. Unfortunately, instead of studying this unexpected and important result, that is, the difference between the amount of shape constancy observed with a circle and a square, Thouless concentrated on the less interesting and already well-known result, which was the fact that shape constancy was not perfect with either shape.

In his second paper (Thouless, 1931b), Thouless performed additional experiments to try to explain the failure of shape constancy he observed. This time he used *only* ellipses, the family of stimuli that, because of its simplicity, is most likely to support the "taking into account" principle. In the first experiment, he tested the effect of reducing cues to depth on the accuracy of shape perception. Accuracy was evaluated by varying the aspect ratio of the ellipse (recall that the aspect ratio of an ellipse is the only parameter characterizing its shape). Three viewing conditions were used: (i) binocular, (ii) binocular through a pseudoscope (a pseudoscope reverses the sign of binocular disparities), and (iii) monocular. The results were as follows: Monocular perception of a slanted ellipse was slightly less accurate than binocular perception. Similarly, binocular (direct) viewing led to somewhat more accurate perception than binocular viewing through a pseudoscope. Based on these results, Thouless concluded (p. 4) that

(i) phenomenal regression in the perception of shapes (i.e., shape constancy) is, at least in a large part, determined by the actual presence of cues to slant (i.e., cues that determine the perceptions of the relative positions of the near and far edges of the ellipse);

(ii) when cues to slant are partially eliminated, shape constancy is reduced.

Thouless considered next which factor (familiarity or availability of depth cues) was responsible for the fact that constancy was *not* eliminated completely by the partial elimination of cues to slant. He considered the following two possibilities: (i) Either the subject was able to use the remaining cues to slant, or (ii) the subject relied on the memory of the actual object (figure).

To decide between these two possibilities, Thouless performed an experiment in which the subject viewed a circle under three slants, producing three different ellipses on the retina. Three viewing conditions were used: (i) binocular with the knowledge that the stimulus shape was a circle, (ii) monocular with the knowledge of the stimulus' shape, and (iii) monocular without the knowledge of the stimulus' shape. Thouless tried to remove all depth cues (except, of course, for binocular disparity, in the case of binocular viewing). In binocular viewing, the perceived aspect ratio was slightly greater than the retinal aspect ratio. In the two monocular conditions, however, the perceived aspect ratio was equal to the retinal aspect ratio. That is, shape constancy completely failed in monocular viewing. This result led Thouless to the following conclusions (p. 7):

(iii) Shape constancy is not dependent on the subject's previous knowledge of the actual shape;

(iv) shape constancy depends only on the presence of cues to slant;

(v) in the presence of cues to slant, the percept is equivalent neither to the retinal image nor to the actual shape of the figure but is a compromise between them.

These five conclusions can be generalized as follows: *Cues to slant are both necessary and sufficient for (approximate) shape constancy.* This statement has been commonly accepted by perceptionists as *the* explanation of shape constancy. It is widely cited in introductory psychology and perception texts. There is, however, a fundamental methodological flaw in Thouless' experiments. Recognizing this flaw drastically changes the conclusions that can be drawn legitimately from Thouless' results.

Thouless used the simplest family of shapes (ellipses), and as has been pointed out repeatedly above, the shape of an ellipse is completely characterized by a single parameter, its aspect ratio. It is also important to remember that a perspective projection of an ellipse is also an ellipse. Furthermore, a perspective projection of any 2D shape on the retina affects the shape with two degrees of freedom for a given retinal position and size (see appendix A, section A.1). From these three facts, *it follows that any ellipse can produce any other ellipse at any given place on the retina.* The family of triangles, which is characterized by only two parameters, is the only other family of shapes for which this statement is true. This statement is not true for any other family of 2D (or 3D) shapes, including a relatively simple family like quadrilaterals, which is characterized by four parameters.

What methodological implication follows from using ellipses to study shape constancy? The answer is simple. *Ellipses must not be used to study shape constancy.* The best way to understand this claim is to begin by assuming that shape constancy is a *problem* that has to be solved by the visual system. Consider first the case of a 2D figure slanted in 3D space (the case of a 3D object will be discussed below). A given 2D figure can produce a large number of different retinal images when the figure is presented with different slants. To solve the shape constancy problem, the observer must recognize that these different retinal images can be produced by the same figure. There is a complementary problem. It is called the "shape ambiguity" problem. In this problem, two or more 2D figures, having different shapes and presented at different slants, produce identical retinal images. The observer's problem is to try to recognize which figure produced a given image. Figure 1.4 illustrates that in the case of ellipses, but not in the case of rectangles (quadrilaterals), shape constancy is confounded with shape ambiguity. It is clear that the only way one can solve the shape ambiguity problem is by taking the slant of the figure into account. In other words, if ellipses are used as stimuli, one is forced to employ a "taking into account" mechanism.[4] Clearly, Thouless' subjects had no choice but to "take slant into account," so it is not surprising that Thouless was able to conclude that this was necessary, but note that he did not realize that his subjects *had* to solve the shape *ambiguity* problem, not the shape *constancy* problem. Once this critical distinction is understood the question is whether his conclusions about the importance of slant generalize to shape constancy when the confound with shape ambiguity is removed by using appropriate stimuli. This issue was neither appreciated nor addressed by Thouless. It is worth noting that shape ambiguity, unlike shape constancy, is probably very rare in everyday life because the shapes of many objects are quite different from each other. To the extent that this is true, it seems unlikely that two (or more) different objects, which are not elliptical or triangular, will give rise to identical retinal images. More than a decade would pass after Thouless published his study before a shape experiment would be published that did not confound shape ambiguity with shape constancy. More than half a century would pass before attention would be called to the problems inherent in Thouless' influential, but misleading, experiments. Most of the intervening experiments on shape contained Thouless' methodological flaw. They tested shape ambiguity rather than shape constancy. All of these studies used either ellipses as stimuli (e.g., Leibowitz & Bourne, 1956; Meneghini & Leibowitz, 1967; Leibowitz, Wilcox, & Post, 1978), triangles as stimuli (e.g., Gottheil & Bitterman, 1951; Beck & Gibson, 1955; Epstein, Bontrager, & Park, 1962; Wallach & Moore, 1962), or trapezoids, chosen in such a way that they were perspectively equivalent (Beck & Gibson, 1955; Kaiser, 1967). Not surprisingly, all of these studies confirmed Thouless' result that cues to slant are necessary and sufficient for solving the *shape ambiguity* problem. These authors, like Thouless, thought, erroneously, that their results were relevant to the phenomenon of shape constancy. They were not.

Shape ambiguity can lead to problems in experiments not only with planar (2D) but also with solid (3D) stimuli (see chapter 4). In fact, confusing shape ambiguity with shape constancy when 3D stimuli are used leads to a further, even more serious problem. Specifically, once shape ambiguity is erroneously assumed to be the same phenomenon as shape constancy, it becomes possible for a researcher to completely change the definition of shape constancy. This actually happened. Recall that shape ambiguity is observed when two or more objects having different shapes produce *the same retinal shape*. Obviously, this is not shape constancy. "Shape constancy" refers to the fact that the percept of the shape of a given object is constant despite *changes in the shape of the object's retinal image, caused by changing the viewing direction* (see endnote 1). In order to solve the shape ambiguity problem, the visual system must make use of information other than the *retinal shape*, as the retinal shape is useless because it is the same for all objects. It provides no useful information whatsoever. Shape constancy is different from shape ambiguity because retinal shape is sufficient to solve the constancy problem. Nothing else is needed. Shape ambiguity is completely different. Retinal shape cannot be used to solve the ambiguity problem, so it is not surprising that concentrating on performing shape ambiguity experiments encouraged studying the efficacy of depth cues, context, and familiarity on the percept of the shape of 3D surfaces. The authors of these experiments mistakenly thought that they were studying shape constancy. They were not. These authors thought that they could study shape constancy by trying to find out whether *perceived shape was constant* when they varied illumination, texture, binocular disparity, context, or familiarity (e.g., Johnston, 1991; Doorschot et al., 2001; Nefs et al., 2005; Scarfe & Hibbard, 2006). However, this approach, keeping viewing direction and thus the *retinal shape* unchanged while varying other properties of the visual stimulus, has nothing to do with shape constancy. This mistake shows that these authors did not realize that they were changing the conventional definition of "shape constancy." It should not be surprising, then, that the results of all of these experiments are not relevant to the study of the well-established phenomenon called "shape constancy." Studying shape constancy requires manipulating the viewing direction, which changes the shape of the test stimuli on the retina. One cannot claim to be studying shape or shape constancy when the viewing direction and the retinal shape of the stimuli are kept constant. Shape ambiguity experiments, in which the viewing direction and the retinal shape of the stimuli are kept constant, like those listed above, can only demonstrate the degree to which depth cues and context provide support for using a "taking slant into account" explanation of a subject's behavior in a shape ambiguity experiment. They have no significance, whatsoever, for understanding shape constancy. Unfortunately, this fact is still not generally appreciated, resulting in considerable confusion in the shape literature. Failure to appreciate the constancy–ambiguity distinction has been one of the major millstones on the road to making progress in the study of shape.

1.5 Stavrianos' (1945) Doctoral Dissertation Was the First Experiment to Show that Subjects Need Not Take Slant into Account to Achieve Shape Constancy

Stavrianos did her dissertation under Woodworth's direction. For most of his career, Woodworth had subscribed to the operation of a "taking into account" mechanism (Woodworth, 1938). When Stavrianos published her dissertation, both experimental results and existing theories implied that the perception of a shape is related to the perception of its orientation. Details of the proposed mechanisms differed among researchers, but it was widely held that there was a relationship between the perceived shape and the orientation of an object. Recall that Thouless (1931a, b) claimed that the percept of the shape of an object depends on the perception of the object's orientation (its slant). Others (Eissler and Klimpfinger—see Stavrianos, 1945) also subscribed to this view, but these authors emphasized that the observer does not have conscious access to the slant of the object. In other words, its orientation is automatically registered and used in determining the perception of shape, but its orientation is not "perceived." This emphasis is closely related to Helmholtz' use of the idea of an unconscious conclusion to "explain" a number of perceptual constancies. One implication of this kind of explanation is that there may be no correlation between the perceived shape and the perceived orientation of an object. Koffka (1935), however, claimed that these two properties of a percept must be correlated: "if two equal retinal shapes give rise to two different perceived shapes, they will at the same time produce the impression that these two shapes are differently oriented" (p. 229). Evidence was available to support Koffka's claim, for example, experiments on size perception showed that cues that affect perceived distance also affect perceived size (e.g., Holway & Boring, 1941). Stavrianos assumed, as Koffka had, that a similar relation would exist between the perceived shape of an object and cues to its slant. She did not know whether to expect an exact, as opposed to an approximate, relation or whether the observer would have conscious access to the percept of slant. Stavrianos designed three experiments to answer these questions. Her subjects were required to make explicit judgments about both the shape and the slant of an object (she used the term "tilt" and "inclination" for what we call "slant"). Her study, specifically her Experiment 1, provides a fundamental contribution to our understanding of shape perception, a contribution that has been largely neglected. A relatively detailed description of Stavrianos' watershed experiment will be provided next. This experiment should have been more influential than it proved to be.

Stavrianos managed to avoid several methodological problems that were inherent in Thouless' experiments. Even though there is good reason to believe that she did not have a full grasp of the differences between the designs of Thouless' and her own experiments (see her discussion of her and Thouless' experiments), she was a much more thorough and systematic experimenter. These admirable traits proved to be critical. On each trial, the subject was presented with a standard rectangle and two comparison rectangles. The comparison rectangles were used to adjust slant and shape to that of the standard rectangle. Specifically, the *slant-variable* rectangle had a constant shape, but its slant could vary. The *shape-variable* rectangle, on the other hand, was always presented in the frontal plane (slant zero), but its shape could vary. The slant of the standard rectangle changed randomly from trial to trial. This rectangle was presented under three "reduction" conditions. Each provided a different number of depth cues. The viewing conditions were (i) normal binocular, (ii) binocular with reduction tubes, and (iii) monocular with a reduction tube. Stavrianos expected, based on preliminary experiments, that reducing cues to depth would substantially harm the accuracy of slant perception. The main question was whether the accuracy of shape perception would deteriorate correspondingly. The subject was asked to adjust first the slant of the slant-variable rectangle and then the aspect ratio of the shape-variable rectangle. By using this order, Stavrianos was trying to facilitate the process of "shape perception by taking slant into account," as would be the case if such a process actually operated in human perception. The adjustments of the slant-variable and shape-variable rectangles were done under normal binocular viewing. The subjects were asked to adjust the shape-variable rectangle so that it represented the "best bet" as to the actual shape of the standard rectangle. She adopted this instruction from Brunswik (1944), who reported that such an "object-directed" attitude leads to the most reliable and accurate results in perceptual constancy experiments.

Stavrianos' Experiment 1, unlike Thouless', did not confound shape constancy with shape ambiguity. That is, her stimuli, rectangles with different shapes, could not produce identical retinal images. This claim follows from the known fact that a single-perspective image of a rectangle, obtained by a calibrated camera (i.e., a camera with known focal length), is sufficient to uniquely reconstruct this rectangle (Perkins & Cooper, 1980, p. 113; Haralick & Shapiro, 1993, volume 2, pp. 80–1). Once this is known, it follows that in Stavrianos' experiment the shape ambiguity problem did not exist. This geometrical fact has a very important implication: It means that *in Stavrianos' experiment, the information about the orientation of the standard rectangle was not needed to match the rectangle's shape accurately; the retinal shape of the rectangle was sufficient to solve the shape constancy problem.*[5]

Note that if Stavrianos had allowed her subjects to adjust more than one parameter of the shape-variable stimulus (as others did—e.g., Kaiser, 1967), she would have introduced the shape ambiguity problem into the experiment and cues to the orientation of shape would have become critical. This follows from the trivial fact that a given retinal image (say, a trapezoid) can be produced by infinitely many different quadrilaterals. Interestingly, it is exactly this aspect of Stavrianos' experiment, that is, eliminating shape ambiguity, that was criticized by others. Gottheil and Bitterman (1951) said that this was a methodological flaw when, in fact, it represented a fundamental improvement over all prior and many subsequent experiments.

Stavrianos first computed correlation coefficients for the relation between the observed error in slant and the error in shape, for each subject and each of the twenty-four experimental conditions used. She found that "no close relation between the deviations for [slant] and for shape is observable for the separate pairs of judgments" (p. 50). She suggested that the relations may have been weak because, within a single reduction condition, the range of errors was not very large. This led her to analyze the accuracy and variability of slant and shape judgments as a function of her three reduction conditions.

The effect of the reduction condition on the mean of slant and shape judgments is shown in her figures 5 and 6 (pp. 52–3). To avoid the confounding effect of day-to-day variability, Stavrianos plotted only means from judgments where a given slant was presented to the subject for all three reduction conditions on the same day. Stavrianos found that reducing cues to depth led to a systematic deterioration in the accuracy of the slant judgments. All differences in the average adjusted slant between the two extreme reduction conditions (normal binocular minus monocular) were positive and substantially larger than the standard errors, indicating that these differences were statistically significant. The direction of the deterioration in accuracy of slant perception was exactly as expected, that is, reducing depth cues led to a greater underestimation of slant.[6] Now, if the percept of shape was based on information about slant, as prior theories and experiments implied, reducing cues to depth should have led to a systematic deterioration of the accuracy of shape judgments. Specifically, the subjects would have been expected to produce smaller aspect ratios in monocular viewing than in normal binocular viewing. This did not happen. The effect of the reduction conditions on the accuracy of shape judgments was small and not systematic.

Next, consider the effect of reducing cues to depth on the variability (precision) of slant and shape judgments. These results are presented in her figures 11 and 12 (pp. 69 and 70), which show that reducing cues to depth led to poorer precision (higher standard deviations) of the slant judgments. Again, this deterioration of slant perception was not accompanied by a corresponding deterioration of shape perception.

These results on the effect of reducing cues to depth on the accuracy and precision of slant and shape perception are the main contribution of Stavrianos. *They clearly show that perceived shape is not systematically related to perceived slant.* This result contradicts both theories of shape perception popular at that time.

Finally, Stavrianos checked whether there is any similarity between the effect of slant on systematic errors in slant judgments and the effect of slant on systematic errors in shape judgments. She found some similarity only in the most extreme case in which viewing was monocular with a reduction tube. She conjectured that shape is one of several cues to slant (p. 65).[7] When other cues are missing, as was presumably the case in monocular viewing, shape remained the only cue. If slant is perceived by taking shape into account, a correlation between shape and slant judgments is expected. It was found. This important observation has been overlooked by all perceptionists until recently (Pizlo, 1994).

To summarize, Stavrianos, in her main experiment, showed that shape constancy does not involve cues to the depth or to the orientation of the figure presented. This result contradicts any theory in which shape constancy depends on context, including all theories of shape perception that claim that perceived shape is based on "taking slant into account." It also contradicts Koffka's claim of an invariant relation between perceived shape and perceived slant. These important implications of Stavrianos' results were overlooked by many perceptionists, including Stavrianos herself (see Hochberg, 1972, for one of very few exceptions). Thouless' results on the perception of ellipses were widely, perhaps even universally, considered to have established the fact that shape constancy requires depth cues. Stavrianos' results clearly contradicted the established wisdom about the relation of shape and slant. However, note that there was actually no contradiction because Thouless had actually studied shape *ambiguity*, showing the trivial fact that information about depth is critical for disambiguating shapes under his conditions. Stavrianos, on the other hand, actually studied shape *constancy*, showing that information about depth is not important for veridicality. Stavrianos' failure to draw appropriate conclusions from her results, and her failure to reject existing shape theories, could be, at least in part, related to the absence of an alternative plausible theory at the time. But at least one thing is clear—namely, that Stavrianos did not understand the nature of the differences between her and Thouless' experiments. This limitation is not as disturbing as one might think because even if she had understood this difference and presented it clearly, progress in the study of shape perception would probably not have been possible in her day.

What alternative theories of shape were available in this period? The philosopher Cassirer (1938) and the mathematicians Courant and Robbins (1941) were the first to conjecture that the perception of shapes from perspective images can be explained by projective invariants (see sections A.2–3).[8] Nothing in her published work suggests that Stavrianos was aware of the idea of geometrical invariants. However, even if she had been, this, in itself, would probably not have led her to propose a new theory of shape constancy because projective (or any other conventional) invariants cannot account for her results. In projective geometry, all rectangles (and in fact all quadrilaterals) are equivalent. It follows that if shape perception were based on projective invariants, all rectangles would have been perceptually equivalent and, thus, Stavrianos, like Thouless, would have ended up studying shape ambiguity, rather than constancy. In short, her results would have been identical to Thouless'! They were very different.[9] In order to explain Stavrianos' results in terms of geometrical invariants, a new class of invariants had to be discovered. These invariants, called "perspective invariants," were first formulated by Pizlo and Rosenfeld (1990, 1992; see section C.9). They can account for existing and new results on shape constancy of 2D figures (Pizlo, 1994). Perspective invariants belong to a more general class of model-based invariants that can be applied to other cases of transformations, which do not form groups (Weinshall, 1993; Rothwell et al., 1993; Pizlo & Loubier, 2000). Thus, Stavrianos was about fifty years ahead of her time. This probably explains why her experiment did not have the influence it deserved.

1.6   Contributions of Gestalt Psychology to Shape Perception (1912–1945)

A great deal of progress toward understanding shape perception has been made since the late 1960s. This progress derived, in large part, from the contributions of the Gestalt psychologists after their work had been incorporated into the Cognitive Revolution. Their main contribution was providing compelling evidence that the perception of shape is produced automatically from the relations among the elements present in the retinal image. They did this by applying what they called the "Laws of Perceptual Organization" (Wertheimer, 1923). The most important of these laws of organization was called "figure–ground organization." It refers to the fact that closed contours establish special closed regions in the percept that correspond to objects in the visual scene. These regions, which were called "figures," are perceived as lying in front of the "background." N.B. that contours always belong to the objects (figures), never to the background. Thus, objects have shapes; backgrounds do not. Figure–ground organization is illustrated in figures 1.2 and 1.3. Clearly, it is easy to see individual objects. They are not confounded with each other or with the background. Furthermore, figure–ground organization is as obvious in the line drawings as in the photographs. Also, note that not only individual objects are seen. The 3D spatial relations within and among the objects are seen, as well. Realize that the 2D image present on your retina when you view figures 1.2 and 1.3 is sufficient to establish veridical 3D percepts of this natural scene. Thus, once the contours of objects are identified in the image, their shapes can be described and then used to solve the shape constancy problem. It will be shown later that the percept of a 3D shape is produced by applying invariants and constraints to the 2D retinal shape. This means that the percept of a 3D shape can be produced only after the contours of the figures have been established. This is why figure–ground organization is so critical. *If the figure–ground organization process fails, invariants and constraints cannot be applied and shape constancy must fail.* This is arguably the most fundamental characteristic of human shape perception. It will be discussed in considerable detail in this book. Unfortunately, the Gestalt psychologists did not elaborate on the relation between shape perception and figure–ground organization. This oversight probably explains why they did not do much to advance the study of shape perception.

The Gestalt psychologists also offered support for their claim that the Laws of Perceptual Organization are innate by showing that one need not learn to perceive such fundamental properties as motion, lightness, or shape. Note that shape, unlike other stimulus properties, is a "Gestalt quality" and, as such, does not depend on the nature of the elements producing it. In fact, the perception of shape, because it is an emergent perceptual property, is arguably the best way to illustrate the uniqueness of the Gestalt contribution to the study of perception. However, Gestalt psychologists, as everyone else at the time, did not appreciate that shape, unlike other perceptual characteristics, has a high degree of complexity. This property permits different shapes to be discriminated easily. Instead of exploring the ways in which shape is special, they concentrated on relational characteristics within the percept, for example, they studied perceived size as a function of perceived distance, and perceived shape as a function of perceived slant. This emphasis on "higher order" variables prevented the Gestalt psychologists from noticing the fundamental problems with Thouless' experiments, an oversight that, in turn, prevented them from rejecting Thouless' "taking slant into account" explanation of shape constancy. Had they appreciated this problem, they might have tried to develop a theory of shape perception based on existing knowledge of projective geometry. Despite this failure, the Gestalt psychologists did pave the way for an explanation of shape perception. Appreciating how they did this requires more than a fleeting discussion of the origin and nature of the Gestalt approach to perception.

The main idea of Gestalt psychology was anticipated by the philosopher Christian von Ehrenfels (1890), who introduced the terminology, as well as the concept, called *Gestaltqualität* (form quality). He pointed out that as soon as there are three elements in the visual field that do not fall on a line, a Gestalt quality emerges, namely, the shape we call "a triangle." The nature, size, or orientation of the three elements does not matter. Once there are three noncollinear elements, a triangle is perceived. If there are four elements, a quadrilateral will be perceived, and so forth. Von Ehrenfels not only pointed this out, and gave this phenomenon the name that was adopted by his students, the Gestalt psychologists, but he also introduced the use of the term "transposition" into the study of perception. This term refers to the fact that a Gestalt quality, such as a triangle, remains when the elements producing it are replaced with other elements or when the elements are translated or rotated. Thus, the properties of the elements composing a shape are not important; only relations among the elements are.

The Gestalt school of perception emphasized these relations and called them "configurations." This is in stark contrast to the Associationists' approach to shape perception. The Associationists emphasized the importance of mental elements they called "sensations." They claimed that the shapes of objects, revealed by the relations among elements, had to be learned by manipulating objects while they were viewed. This claim was at the center of the Gestalt psychologists' attack on the Associationists represented by Helmholtz' student Wilhelm Wundt and his English-speaking student Edward Bradford Titchener, who led the Associationist approach in Europe and in America when Max Wertheimer launched the Gestalt Revolution in 1912 (see Heidbreder, 1933, for a good description of these "schools of psychology" and their controversies). Koffka, one of the three founding "fathers" of the Gestalt Revolution called the Associationists' rejection of the possibility of relations (interactions) among elements in the retinal image the "constancy hypothesis." In his words, this hypothesis *"implies that all locally stimulated excitations run their course without regard to other excitations"* (Koffka, 1935, pp. 96–7).[10]

Gestalt psychologists contributed another idea that occupies a prominent place in contemporary research on shape perception, specifically, they placed emphasis on the importance of simplicity in determining the nature of a given percept. Their simplicity principle is analogous to what is called "a minimum principle" in physics. They embodied their simplicity principle in their Law of Prägnanz (*Prägnanz* in German means "succinctness, conciseness, or terseness"). Koffka (1935, p. 110) described this law as follows: *"perceptual organization is always as good as the prevailing conditions allow,"* where good means regular, symmetrical, or simple. An example illustrating the operation of this simplicity principle is shown in figure 1.6. Here, at least two different interpretations are possible. One is a pair of vertical lines with a symmetrical figure between them. The other is a superposition of the letters *M* and *W*. The letters are superimposed in such a way that parts of the *M* and parts of the *W* form longer, continuous lines and a closed form. Despite our familiarity with the letters *M* and *W*, and indeed, despite our knowledge that this interpretation is possible, it is much easier and more natural to see two longer lines and a closed figure between them than the letters *M* and *W* (after Koffka, 1935, p. 155). The "good figure" prevails. The Gestalt psychologists called the perceptual organizing principles responsible for this result "good continuation" and "closure."

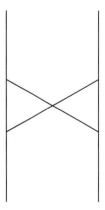

Figure 1.6
It is not easy to see the letters *M* and *W*. Good continuation and symmetry lead to a different (simpler) perceptual organization (after Koffka, 1935).

The Gestalt psychologists also introduced a number of other ideas that influenced subsequent theories of shape perception in more indirect ways, for example, Blum's (1973) symmetry axes and "grassfire" model, Grossberg's (Grossberg & Mingolla, 1985) neural network model, and Ginsburg's (1986) spatial filter model. All of these approaches derive from simple assumptions about relationships between the nature of the percept and its underlying physiological cause. The Gestalt psychologists took this on very early in the development of their theory. Their interest is embodied in what they called "psychophysiological isomorphism." For example, if one perceives an object as moving, one could claim, as Wertheimer (1912) did, that the underlying brain process consists of moving excitation within the brain tissue.[11] Gestalt psychologists claimed that the relations between the percept and its physiological correlate were topological, not metric. That is, only neighborhood relations are preserved; the distances between elements are not. Gestalt psychologists embodied their isomorphism principle in an electrical brain currents model. Specifically, a minimum state of the brain currents was supposed to provide a physiological explanation of the simplicity principle responsible for perceptual organization (Köhler, 1920). Köhler, who was the third founding father of Gestalt psychology, made extensive use of the simplicity principle in developing the concept of psychophysiological isomorphism. He had a background not only in psychology but also in physics and mathematics. He was quite familiar with the use of a minimum principle, the kind of principle that allowed elegant formulations of laws in physics (Lanczos, 1970). For example, the Fermat principle, according to which light travels along the path that *minimizes* the time of travel,[12] allows derivation of the laws of reflection and refraction in optics. Another example is Kirchhoff's laws for electrical circuits, that is, given a circuit with a voltage source and resistors, the currents in the branches of the circuit will be such that the total amount of heat generated in the resistors is *minimal*. According to Köhler, similar simplicity mechanisms were likely to apply in perception. For Köhler, the steady state of electrical brain currents was a plausible physiological counterpart (a cause) of perceptual simplicity (Köhler, 1920). Köhler's claims, which may seem far-fetched to many today, fitted in well with the zeitgeist of his time. We are now sure that electrical brain currents do not provide a plausible physiological model of perception as Köhler proposed, but in his day, such speculations were quite reasonable.[13] The Gestalt psychologists' insistence on the importance of inherited, built-in, perceptual organizing principles and on simplicity constraining the nature of perceptual organization continue to be important. Next, we will consider how their simplicity principle fared following its introduction.

1.6.1 The Role of Simplicity in the Perception of Shape

If we accept the claim that the simplicity principle is critical in determining the percept, it becomes important to know what we mean by "simplicity." It is one thing to state that a given percept is simple, after the percept has been observed, and quite another to predict what the percept will be like before it occurs. A precise formulation of simplicity was not available until information theory was formulated by Shannon in 1948. Until then, attempts to provide a Gestalt-inspired theory of shape perception were doomed to fail despite the fact that the Gestalt emphasis on inbuilt automatic perceptual organizing processes had promise. Their attempts to develop a theory of shape perception will be illustrated by describing how Koffka dealt with the fundamental question about shape first posed by Wertheimer in 1923.

1.6.1.1 Why Do Things Look as They Do   Koffka's (1935) approach to perception, in general, and to shape perception, in particular, begins by raising this question (p. 75). He discusses two commonsensical answers: (i) Things look as they do because they are what they are, and (ii) things look as they do because their retinal images are what they are. Neither answer is accepted by Koffka, who turns next to the answer proposed by the Associationists, who held that the nature of the percept is determined by an unconscious conclusion in which learning and associations play the crucial role. Koffka does not accept this empiristic answer on the grounds that it does not offer an adequate explanation of the fact that human and animal infants, who have had very little time for learning, demonstrate many perceptual constancies.

Koffka's "true answer" to his question "Why do things look as they do?" is that things look as they do because this is the simplest interpretation of their retinal image (p. 98). Koffka's answer begs the question because he could not provide a formal operational definition of simplicity. This forced him to speculate about the physiological basis of simplicity. He did this by invoking what the Gestalt psychologists called "field forces." These forces were associated with the electrical activities of the brain. The brain field, according to Koffka, involves the operation of two forces, one internal and one external. The external force is produced by the proximal stimulus (the retinal image). The internal force is produced by the brain's tendency toward simple percepts. Each force is represented by electrical brain currents whose steady state (the minimum state) is the physiological correlate of the percept. The two forces interact. If both forces act in the same direction, as would presumably be the case when the retinal image is simple— for example, a circle—the percept is stable. When the two forces are in strong conflict, as would be the case when the retinal image is an irregular shape, the percept should be unstable (Koffka, 1935, pp. 138–9). For Gestalt psychologists, the circle was special. It was the simplest, most regular shape. It was the simplest 2D shape because the given surface area was enclosed by the minimal-length, therefore simplest, contour. In other words, the circle is the most "compact" 2D figure, because a contour of a given length encloses the maximal area. This property of "compactness" will take on considerable significance later when we move to consideration of 3D shapes, where a sphere will become the simplest figure. An example of a simplicity principle operating in three dimensions can be illustrated by a soap bubble: A soap bubble will always take on a spherical shape because a sphere requires the minimum amount of energy to maintain its integrity. Note that it is difficult to demonstrate the operation of a simplicity (minimum) principle with 2D shapes, the case most often discussed by Koffka (1935). Koffka, and others who were sympathetic to Gestalt ideas, had little success when they tried to demonstrate the operation of a minimum principle by measuring absolute thresholds of 2D shapes. It is much easier to demonstrate the application of a minimum principle with 3D shapes. This is how it can be done.

1.6.1.2 Perception of 3D Shape from 2D Images   *Koffka's treatment of the perception of 3D shapes from 2D images begins with the following statement:* "three-dimensional shapes are matters of organization in the same way as two-dimensional ones, depending on the same kind of laws" (p. 161). *What Koffka is saying is that 3D percepts, like 2D percepts, derive from built-in automatic organizing processes. They do not depend on learning. The 3D percept, like the 2D percept, reflects the operation of a simplicity principle.* He supports this claim with a discussion of Kopfermann's (1930) and Schriever's (1925)

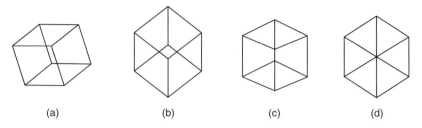

(a)   (b)   (c)   (d)

Figure 1.7
Kopfermann's stimuli (from Kopfermann, 1930, p. 298, figure 1—with kind permission of Springer Science and Business Media).

experiments. They studied 2D representations of solid objects whose percepts were "simpler" when they were viewed as 3D objects.

Kopfermann used a set of orthographic projections of a cube. The subjects were shown line drawings like those in figure 1.7. The four figures are different with respect to regularity or simplicity as measured by topological and metric properties. Specifically, these figures differ with respect to the number of points of intersection of the lines contained in each figure, as well as with respect to the lengths of their line segments and the sizes of their angles. The subjects in Kopfermann's (1930) study were asked whether they saw a 2D (planar) figure or a 3D (solid) object. The figures in (c) and (d) usually led to the percept of a planar (flat) figure, identical with the figure itself. The figures in (a) and (b), on the other hand, usually led to the percept of a cube.[14] These observations allowed her to conclude that the percept is equivalent to the 2D projection when this projection is simple as in (c) and (d). However, when the 2D projection is more complex, as in (a) and (b), the "simpler" 3D object is seen. In fact, the percept produced by (a) or (b) corresponds to a cube, the most symmetrical 3D object consistent with these figures' retinal images. This fits nicely with Koffka and his Gestalt colleagues' conjectures about the important role of simplicity in shape perception. Note also that, as Koffka pointed out, the percept in figure 1.7a corresponds to a 3D regular (simple) figure despite a powerful conflicting cue (external force), namely, binocular disparity, which should tell the observer that the stimulus is actually flat (Koffka, 1935, p. 161).

A related experiment was performed by Schriever in 1925 (see Koffka, 1935, pp. 274–5). He used a meaningless 3D object (figure 1.8) composed of three connected bars located in different depth planes. He then

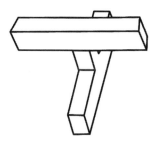

Figure 1.8
Schriever's stimulus (after Koffka, *Principles of Gestalt psychology*, Harcourt Brace 1935, figure 82, p. 274—with kind permission of the publisher).

introduced a conflict between binocular disparity and perceptual organization of the meaningless 3D object's retinal image. He did this by photographing the object from slightly different viewing directions and then using a stereoscope to reverse the bar's order in depth by presenting the left image to the right eye and the right image to the left eye. If the binocular percept of this 3D meaningless object were determined by binocular disparity, the subject should have perceived the parts of the object with their order in depth reversed. Instead, the subject perceived the depth order given by the available monocular perceptual grouping principles, namely, good continuation and occlusion. Binocular disparity had little, if any, effect. This is a nice example of the way Gestalt psychologists determined the relative importance of various cues and rules of perceptual organization. Here, good continuation (internal force) was found to be more important than binocular disparity (external force). Another way of stating Schriever's result is to say that *the perceived 3D shape had more to do with the 2D shape on the retina than with the depth relations indicated by binocular disparity.*

The Gestalt psychologists did not say much more about the perception of 3D shape produced by 2D retinal images than described above. This is unfortunate because the relation between a percept of a 3D object and its 2D retinal image is critical, especially when the role of a simplicity principle in shape perception is considered. Once the 2D shape on the retina is established through the operation of figure–ground organization, the simplicity principle is involved in producing the 3D shape percept. The simplicity principle is not needed to *simplify* the percept of the 2D retinal shape. It follows that invocation of a simplicity principle is not (i) needed or (ii) productive when one confines discussion to the perception of 2D (planar) shapes, which are abstractions. N.B., *there are no 2D objects, no matter how thin.* Unfortunately, this canon has not been and is not widely appreciated, an oversight that has led to a great many pointless experiments, controversies, and erroneous conclusions. Its neglect has been as big an obstacle to the development of an adequate theory of shape as Thouless' naiveté with respect to the projective properties of triangles and ellipses proved to be in the study of shape constancy.

1.6.1.3 Studies of Shape Thresholds The interest in shape thresholds was initiated by Goethe, who reported that an afterimage of a square becomes more and more circular with the passage of time (Koffka, 1935, p. 143). Koffka made note of this and went on to claim that internal forces, which bias a percept toward simplicity, compete with external forces produced by the square because it is not as simple as the "simplest form," that is, a circle. In other words, the afterimage of the square weakens over time and the resulting percept becomes more distorted in the direction of greater simplicity. It comes to be perceived more and more like the simpler, "best," figure, the circle.

Gestalt psychologists used several methods to test the conflict between internal and external forces by using (i) short exposure times, (ii) low contrast stimuli, (iii) small targets, and (iv) afterimages. These methods were believed to provide a means of studying how competition between internal and external forces determined the percept. In other words, these methods allowed them to study the relative importance of the simplicity principle vis-à-vis properties of the retinal image.

Studying weak external forces lends itself naturally to the measurement of both detection and identification thresholds. The main prediction of the Gestalt theory was that simple shapes would be easier to detect and identify than complex shapes. This line of research led to a large number of studies published over the span of more than four decades, beginning in the early 1920s. The interested reader should consult reviews by Hochberg (1972, pp. 443–4), who was involved in this research himself, and also Zusne (1970, pp. 265–9, 304–7), who was not. The results are, at best, inconclusive: (i) Decreasing the "strength" of the stimulus does not necessarily lead to simpler percepts, (ii) the luminance threshold for detecting shapes does not depend systematically on the nature of the shape itself, and (iii) complex shapes do not necessarily require longer exposure duration for successful shape identification. Today, no one studies shape thresholds. This is not because the questions leading to these experiments have been answered, but because these experiments have not been productive. These experiments were based on an implausible assumption, namely, that the percept arises from a conflict between simplicity constraints and properties of the retinal image. This kind of psychodynamical approach has fallen out of favor. We now make a quite different assumption, namely, that *the simplicity principle is incorporated in perceptual mechanisms in order to make up for information lost due to (i) the projection from the distal to the proximal stimulus and (ii) the presence of noise in the visual system.* This assumption leads to different kinds of experiments than those performed by the Gestalt psychologists (see section 4.3).

To summarize, the Gestalt psychologists' preference for studying 2D shapes, as well as their commitment to their physiological model of Prägnanz, did not produce useful results on shape perception beyond the work of Kopfermann and Schriever. The Gestalt psychologists, as well as everyone else until recently, simply did not appreciate the fact that the only way to study the role of simplicity in shape perception is to use 3D objects (or 2D images of 3D objects). Stimuli with only two dimensions are too impoverished to reveal how simplicity constraints can compensate for information lost in the projection from distal to proximal stimulus. Gestalt psychologists were on the right track in emphasizing the role of simplicity in perception, but they failed to provide a formal definition of what they meant by "simplicity." Obviously, they cannot be faulted for failing to do so because information theory, the theory which deals with the concept of simplicity, was not formulated until 1948 (Shannon, 1948). A revival of the Gestalt approach took place in the early 1950s. This revival was stimulated by the formulation of information theory and by the shift of emphasis from research with 2D shapes to research with 3D shapes. Once these were in place, it became possible to make major advances in the study of perception and cognition. These changes led to what had been called the "Cognitive Revolution."

2 The Cognitive Revolution Leads to Neo-Gestaltism and Neo-Empiricism

Progress in science and technology made during World War II contributed a lot to what has been called the "Cognitive Revolution" (Neisser, 1967; Gardner, 1987). The formulation of the theory and design of computers led the way (Turing, 1936; von Neuman, 1951). Computers allowed the manipulation of both numbers and symbols. This opened up the possibility of writing computer programs that could perform such important human tasks as pattern recognition, the coding and decoding of messages, game playing, and problem solving (Feigenbaum & Feldman, 1963; Minsky, 1968). Another element that contributed significantly to the Cognitive Revolution was called "cybernetics" (Wiener, 1948). Cybernetics provided unified treatments of (i) engineering systems that make use of negative feedback (Craik, 1943; Mayr, 1970; Bennett, 1979, 1993), (ii) biological systems designed to achieve homeostasis (Cannon, 1932; Ashby, 1940), and (iii) ecological systems based on prey–predator relations (Lotka, 1925), as well as (iv) purposive goal-directed behavior of both human beings and animals (Münsterberg, 1914; Warren, 1916; Tolman, 1932; Hull, 1930, 1937).[1] Wiener, the founder of cybernetics, actually went so far as to say that cybernetics is the branch of engineering that deals with designing "teleological systems" (Rosenblueth, Wiener, & Bigelow, 1943). Once cybernetics is described in this way, one might be led to claim that cybernetics demystifies the philosophical concept called "teleology" by showing that the concept of a "final cause" *is actually acceptable* in science and engineering after all. This claim goes much too far. "Final causes" still do not have a place in science and probably never will. Making a claim like this requires changing the meaning of the word "teleology." In philosophy, "teleology" means that the *present* can be affected by the *future*. In cybernetics, it means that the *present* can be affected by a *model* (representation or expectation) of the *future*, not by the future itself.

The third element that contributed to the Cognitive Revolution was the formulation of information theory (Shannon, 1948). Information theory grew out of several disciplines, namely, statistics, communication, and control engineering (Cherry, 1978). The fourth element was neuroscience, which studies the anatomy and physiology of the nervous system, particularly of the brain (Talbot & Marshall, 1941; McCulloch & Pitts, 1943; Kuffler, 1953; Hubel & Wiesel, 1962). Neuroscience played an important role in the Cognitive Revolution, often overshadowing the importance of the other three elements (Jeffress, 1951; Hebb, 1949). However, the contribution of neuroscience to our understanding of human shape perception has been rather modest. The other three elements have been much more important to date.

In psychology, the beginnings of the Cognitive Revolution were closely related to the first and third elements, that is, the development of computer science and the formulation of information theory. Specifically, psychologists began to count "bits of information" contained in linguistic messages (Shannon, 1948; Miller & Selfridge, 1950; Miller, 1951), in sensorimotor channels (Hick, 1952; Fitts, 1954), in short-term memory (Miller, 1956), and in the perception of patterns (Attneave, 1954, 1959). It was hardly counterintuitive that messages and patterns that were *simpler* and had greater redundancy would be easier to code, respond to, memorize, and recognize. No one was surprised when this proved to be the case. It quickly became apparent that information theory offered the possibility for a precise quantitative formulation of the Gestalt Law of Prägnanz (e.g., Attneave, 1954). This development inspired what will be called the "neo-Gestalt" movement. This movement was led by Julian Hochberg, Fred Attneave, David Perkins, and Hans Wallach. Their most important contributions will be described next.

2.1 Hochberg's Attempts to Define Simplicity Quantitatively

2.1.1 The Role of the Simplicity Principle in Determining Whether a Shape Will Be Perceived in Two or in Three Dimensions

An influential paper by Hochberg and McAlister (1953) started a series of studies aimed at defining the Gestalt simplicity principle operationally.

These authors began by replicating Kopfermann's experiment, published in German in 1930 and described by Koffka in 1935, with 2D stimuli that were perceived as "simpler" when they were perceived as 3D objects. They improved the methodology and interpreted their results using the language, but not the formalisms, of information theory. The 2D stimuli they used are shown in figure 2.1. Each of the four stimuli can lead either to a 2D percept analogous to the drawing itself or to a 3D percept, namely, a cube.[2] The complexity of the 3D interpretation was the same for all four stimuli because only one 3D interpretation was perceived, namely, a cube. However, the complexity of the 2D interpretation was different for each of the four stimuli shown in this figure. Hochberg and McAlister proposed that the "complexity" of a stimulus should be measured by the amount of information that is needed to describe the stimulus. This led them to a reformulation of Kopfermann's claim about the relation between the simplicity of an interpretation and the likelihood of a given percept. Hochberg and McAlister's hypothesis was that "the less the amount of information needed to define a given [perceptual] organization, . . . the more likely that the figure will be . . . perceived [as 2D or 3D]" (p. 361). Hochberg and McAlister proposed three geometrical features that can be used to measure the complexity of a figure, namely, the number of (i) line segments, (ii) angles, and (iii) points of intersection (junctions). For example, stimulus (c) in figure 2.1 has thirteen line segments, twenty angles, and eight junction points.[3] According to the authors' classification, (a) and (b) are equally complex, (c) is simpler, and (d) is the simplest. Therefore, (d) should be perceived as a 2D pattern, whereas (a) and (b) should be perceived as a cube.

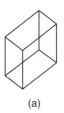 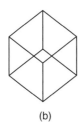 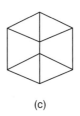 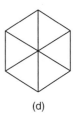

(a)   (b)   (c)   (d)

Figure 2.1
Stimuli used by Hochberg and McAlister (1953). Stimulus (d) is simple when perceived as a 2D figure. Stimulus (a) is complex when perceived as a 2D figure but simple when perceived as a "cube" (from Hochberg & McAlister, 1953).

Hochberg and McAlister (1953) estimated the likelihood of perceiving a 2D versus a 3D interpretation as follows: The subject viewed each figure for 100 seconds. During this period, thirty-three tones were presented at random intervals. The subject was asked to report the interpretation (2D or 3D) perceived when each tone was heard. The frequency of 2D interpretations was computed. Eighty subjects were tested with each of the four stimuli. The relative frequencies of 2D interpretations based on all eighty subjects were as follows: 1.3%, 0.7%, 49% and 60% for stimuli (a), (b), (c), and (d), respectively, confirming, the authors' prediction.

These results are consistent with the authors' hypothesis that simpler interpretations, that is, the interpretations that require less information, are preferred perceptually. Note that Hochberg and McAlister (1953) did not actually compute the amount of information quantitatively by counting bits. Instead, they used quantitative measures that correspond intuitively, rather than formally, to the amount of information. For example, according to Hochberg and McAlister, a quadrilateral is more complex (requires more information to describe) than a triangle. No one would question this classification, but it is important to realize that counting angles is not equivalent to counting bits. Could Hochberg and McAlister have improved their "theory" by actually using the number of bits required to describe a figure as a measure of complexity of the figure's shape? I doubt it. There were a number of attempts to do this (e.g., Leeuwenberg, 1971), but none of them were successful. Specifically, each theory could "explain" the percepts for only a very limited set of stimuli. The main reason for these failures was that these theories were based on an implausible assumption, namely, that the goal of the visual system is to produce *simple percepts*. It is more reasonable to assume that the goal of the visual system is to produce *veridical percepts*. Constraints, such as simplicity, are tools that can be used to achieve this goal. The change of emphasis from the simplicity to the veridicality of the percept did not take place until the machine vision community entered the field in the 1970s.

In a follow-up study, Hochberg and Brooks (1960) set out to determine whether the simplicity principle applies to a wider range of objects (polyhedra) and whether it can predict the results of new psychophysical experiments rather than simply account for data already collected. In their first experiment, line drawings of nine polyhedra were used. For each polyhe-

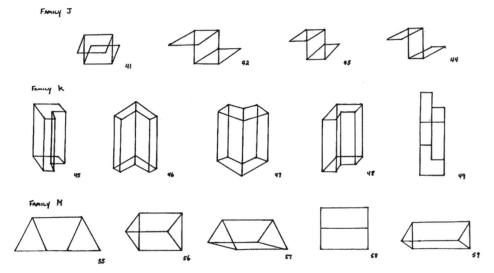

Figure 2.2
Three "families" of shapes (*J*, *K*, and *M*) used by Hochberg and Brooks (1960). (From *American Journal of Psychology*. Copyright 1960 by the Board of Trustees of the University of Illinois. Used with permission of the University of Illinois Press and of the authors.)

dron, they constructed four or five figures, each figure representing a different view of the same object. The views produced by a given polyhedron formed what the authors called a "family," corresponding to a given polyhedron (figure 2.2 shows three such families). Four hundred thirty naive subjects were asked to rate the apparent tridimensionality of each figure using a graphical scale ranging from 0 to 10. The authors considered seventeen features that could be related to the complexity of a 2D figure, like the number of angles, the number of junction points, and so forth. Then, they computed correlations between all pairs of features, as well as the figure's perceived tridimensionality. They factor analyzed the resulting correlation matrix and chose three features that accounted for a large proportion of the variance in their results. These features were (i) total number of interior angles, (ii) total number of continuous line segments (i.e., ignoring intersections), and (iii) total number of different angles divided by the total number of angles. Then, they computed a regression model describing the effect of these three features on the degree of tridimensionality perceived.

In their second experiment, Hochberg and Brooks (1960) tested how well this regression model could predict perceived tridimensionality with line drawings produced by new polyhedra. The correlation between the subjects' ratings and the predictions of their regression model was very high, .98, clearly allowing them to claim that their model had high predictive power. Finally, the authors verified the generality of their results with a different scaling method. They used the paired-comparison method to rank order the apparent tridimensionality of the figures. The rank order obtained agreed closely with the order derived from the magnitude estimation procedure used in the second experiment. This strongly suggested that the high correlations between human judgments and model predictions are not restricted to a single psychophysical method.

2.1.2 The Role of Learning in Shape Perception

Having established that monocular shape perception, specifically the perception of shapes of 3D objects from their 2D images, involves a simplicity principle, Hochberg and Brooks (1962) went on to find out whether learning plays an important role in shape perception. The Gestalt psychologists, who emphasized the role of simplicity in perception, were nativists. According to them, the rules of perceptual organization were innate. It seemed that if one wanted to show that nativism cannot be the full story, and that learning after birth is needed to form perceptual mechanisms, the perception of objects from pictures would be the best place to start. The reason is simple. There were not very many pictures of objects in the natural environment during the early evolution of human beings. Pictures have become common only in relatively recent human history, probably not extending back much more than 50,000 years. It seems unlikely that the perceptual ability to see and recognize 3D scenes from 2D pictures and line drawings has had sufficient time to establish itself in our genes. Obviously, if one were able to demonstrate the absence of a need for learning in recognizing 3D objects in 2D pictures, one would have made quite a strong argument in favor of the nativistic position.

The fact that pictures of 3D scenes are devoid of many useful depth cues, such as binocular disparity, motion parallax, accommodation, and vergence cues, all of which are present when we view 3D scenes, suggested to some (e.g., Gibson, 1950) that experiments involving pictures could never reveal how the visual system operates in natural, ecologically valid situations. Those who believed this argued that pictures should not be used to study perception because results obtained in experiments with pictures (such as Hochberg and McAlister's, 1953) would not generalize to ecologically valid, full-cue conditions. Specifically, according to Gibson, no a priori rules of organization are needed when real 3D scenes are viewed. Perceptual rules of organization become important only when impoverished stimuli, such as pictures, are used (Gibson, 1950, p. 196). Gibson's claim provided a second reason motivating Hochberg and Brooks' (1962) study.

A newly born baby boy served as the subject in this experiment. As his language skills were developing during his first two years, he was exposed to many common objects and toys and taught the names of these objects, but he was prevented from seeing 2D representations of such objects to the extent this was possible. He was not allowed to see either movies or still pictures. Hochberg and Brooks expected that the child would be able to recognize familiar objects and be able to name them. The experimental question was whether the child could also name the objects when presented with pictures of these objects. The training phase of the experiment lasted for only nineteen months because by this time the child could no longer be prevented from seeing pictures without interfering with his normal development and with normal family life. The second phase of the experiment consisted of two tests. Twenty-one pictures were used in the first test. Photographs of objects and line drawings of these objects were included in the test. The child's responses were tape-recorded as these stimuli were presented one at a time. After this first test, the child was exposed to many picture books in order to facilitate "perceptual learning." A second test with nineteen new pictures of objects was administered after a month of such perceptual learning.

The child had almost no difficulty in naming familiar objects from pictures in both the first and second test. This result clearly shows that a single 2D image of a particular 3D object had produced a 3D percept in the boy's mind. Furthermore, this percept must have been very similar (possibly even identical) to the percept resulting from viewing the actual 3D object. Note that performance on the first test was as good as performance on the second test. These results strongly suggest that *perceiving 3D objects from 2D pictures is innate and that this perceptual ability involves the same mechanisms as perceiving real 3D objects*. Finally, now that we know that perceiving

3D objects from 2D images does involve a priori simplicity constraints, it becomes possible to claim that *the simplicity constraints that are used to perceive 3D objects are used to perceive 3D objects from 2D pictures, as well.* Once this is appreciated it becomes clear that Gibson's claim was unwarranted. Theories of perception based on studies of the perception of 3D objects from 2D pictures *are* actually quite relevant for studying the perception of real objects.

2.2   Attneave's Experiment on 3D Shape

Attneave (1959) pointed out that the Cognitive Revolution raised two new important questions, namely, (i) what was the maximum transmission rate and (ii) how much information can be transmitted through sensory and motor communication channels (p. 43). These questions do not actually apply to the perception of 3D shapes. Transmitting information through a communication channel deals primarily with a one-to-one mapping, while the perception of 3D shapes deals with a one-to-many mapping from the 2D proximal stimulus to the 3D percept. Attneave's early research concentrated on 2D stimuli and their corresponding 2D percepts (Attneave, 1954, 1959). By doing this, he was able to apply the communication framework to his theory of perception. Note, however, that this approach could not work with the kind of 2D stimuli that produce a 3D percept, for example, the kind of stimuli used in Hochberg and McAlister's (1953) study. In 1959, Attneave apparently underestimated the significance of Hochberg and McAlister's contribution. It took him ten years before he switched his emphasis from the perception of 2D shapes to the perception of 3D shapes (Attneave & Frost, 1969).

Hochberg and his associates had demonstrated that the simplicity of the retinal image determines whether the percept will be 2D or 3D. This showed that there was a relation between the simplicity and the topological properties of the percept. Attneave and Frost (1969) took the next step by demonstrating that the simplicity of the object and its retinal image determine the Euclidean properties of the 3D percept, such as the orientation of the edges of a polyhedron. Their subjects simultaneously viewed a line drawing of a polyhedron monocularly and a rod in 3D binocularly. They were asked to adjust the orientation of the rod so that it matched the perceived orientation of the edges of the polyhedron. Three different images were used: (i) an orthographic image of a rectangular parallelepiped (a parallelepiped is a 3D prism whose faces are all parallelograms; a rectangular parallelepiped is a parallelepiped whose trihedral angles are all right angles), (ii) an orthographic image of a cube, and (iii) a perspective image of a cube (figure 2.3). The perspective image was computed assuming that the line of sight was orthogonal to the picture plane at the vertex of the Y junction of the line drawing, and that the viewing distance was 47 cm, the distance from which the subjects actually viewed the pictures.

Now, consider the logic behind Attneave and Frost's experiment. If the visual system maximizes the simplicity of the 3D perceptual interpretation, a perspective image of a cube will lead to the percept of a cube because a cube is the simplest 3D interpretation of the image of a cube. Furthermore, it is reasonable to expect that the perceived cube will have the same 3D orientation as the cube that was used to compute the perspective image. The orientation of a cube can be "measured" by the orientations of the edges of the cube relative to the frontal plane. Thus, it seems plausible that the perceived orientation of a cube can be measured by measuring the perceived orientation of its edges. The authors derived a formula that determines the orientation of the edges of a cube from the image of the cube. They limited their analysis of these geometrical relations to the three edges forming a Y junction. Consider figure 2.4 and the 3D orientation ϕ_1 of edge L_1 (whose image is l_1) relative to the frontal plane. This

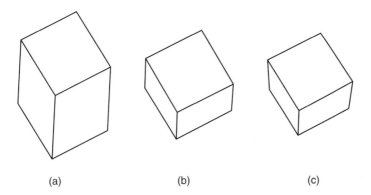

(a)   (b)   (c)

Figure 2.3
Stimuli used by Attneave and Frost (1969): (a) is an orthographic image of a rectangular parallelepiped, (b) is an orthographic image of a cube, and (c) is a perspective image of a cube (with kind permission of the Psychonomic Society Publications).

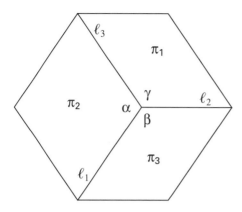

Figure 2.4
Orthographic image of a cube. Angles α, β, and γ satisfy Perkins' law, that is, all
three are obtuse in this orthographic image.

angle can be computed from the following formula (Attneave & Frost's
equation 13):

$$\sin(\phi_1) = \frac{1}{\sqrt{\tan \alpha \cdot \tan \beta}}.$$ (2.1)

Note that this formula applies not only to an orthographic but also to a
perspective image of the Y junction of a cube, as long as the line connecting the center of projection and the vertex of this junction is orthogonal
to the image plane.

How could this equation (2.1) be used to test the role of simplicity in
shape perception? The authors' reasoning was as follows. If the subject
perceives a cube, the subject's judgments of ϕ_1 should conform to equation
(2.1). Now, look at figure 2.3b, which was produced by an orthographic
projection of a cube. In a perspective projection, the edges of a cube that
are farther from the observer project to shorter line segments. This is illustrated in figure 2.3c, which is a valid perspective image of a cube. The other
two images, (a) and (b), cannot be produced by a cube in a perspective
projection and, thus, do not allow for such a perceptual interpretation.
The authors adopted (apparently after Hochberg & McAlister, 1953) a
qualitative model, in which there are only two possible interpretations: a
cube (the 3D interpretation) and a flat figure identical to the line drawing
presented. In all three figures (figure 2.3a–c), the Y junction is consistent
with a cube interpretation. In both (b) and (c), but not in (a), the projected

lengths of the Y junction are consistent with a cube interpretation. Finally, in (c), but not in (a) or (b), the remaining angles of the figure, as well as the lengths of the remaining edges, are consistent with a cube interpretation. Attneave and Frost assumed that the two different interpretations (3D and 2D) conflict with each other and that the conflict results in a combination (fusion) of the two interpretations.[4] Thus, the subject's judgment should be closest to that predicted by equation (2.1) in case (c), and farthest from that prediction in case (a). This is indeed what happened. The slope of the regression line for the relation between the perceived ϕ (dependent variable) and computed ϕ, was 0.34, 0.59, and 0.63 for images (a), (b), and (c), respectively.

Now, consider theoretical issues that follow directly from Attneave and Frost's (1969) study. First, consider the relation between the perceived shape and the perceived 3D orientation (slant), the issue discussed at length earlier. Attneave and Frost used 2D line drawings. Therefore, the stimulus itself did not provide any conventional cues to the slant of the edges or faces, like shading, texture, motion, or binocular disparity. In fact, the edges and faces were perceived as having 3D orientations *only because* they were perceived as part of a 3D object. Clearly, in the case of line drawings, the percept of a 3D shape cannot be based on the percept of the 3D orientations of its edges or faces. The particular 3D percept is obtained by the application of a simplicity principle to the 3D shape. For example, the percept produced by images such as figure 2.3c can be obtained by making all angles equal (here equal to 90 deg) or by choosing a 3D object with the maximal volume for a given surface area (i.e., maximal compactness). The percept of the 3D orientations of the edges and faces of the 3D object does not precede, but rather is preceded by, the percept of the object's shape. In other words, the shape is perceived before its edges are perceived. Prior theorists studying shape constancy concentrated exclusively on a "shape from slant" explanation, but as was shown in chapter 1, another explanation, namely, "slant from shape," is more likely to be appropriate. Attneave and Frost's (1969) experiment provided converging evidence for such an explanation.

2.3   Perkins' Contribution: Emphasis Shifts from Simplicity to Veridicality

Perkins' experiments were stimulated by the work of the "Transactional psychologists," who emphasized the importance of Ames' distorted room

(Ittelson, 1968; Kilpatrick, 1961). Perkins was the first to appreciate the relation between the work of Ames' group and the work of the Gestalt and neo-Gestalt psychologists (Kopfermann, 1930; Hochberg and McAlister, 1953; Attneave and Frost, 1969). By bringing these two traditions together, Perkins made a good case for the suggestion that simplicity and likelihood principles are conceptually closely related in the sense that "good form is a good bet" (Perkins, 1976; see also Mach, 1906, who made this suggestion earlier). Perkins was also the first to show that shape constraints can predict the 3D shape percept. Recall that Hochberg and McAlister (1953) were only able to explain the role of constraints in determining whether the percept would be 2D or 3D. Attneave and Frost (1969) were only able to explain (to some degree) the role of constraints in the perceived 3D orientations of the edges of an object. Perkins took the next step by bringing together constraints and the 3D shape percept. Perkins, by doing this, anticipated the way 3D shape perception is studied and modeled today. An additional important aspect of Perkins' work was his insistence on understanding the geometrical relation between the distal and proximal stimulus. Understanding this relation is often (one might even say, always) critical for interpreting the results of a psychophysical experiment on shape perception.

2.3.1 Rectangular versus Nonrectangular Parallelepipeds

In his first study, Perkins (1972) tested subjects' ability to identify rectangular and nonrectangular boxes (parallelepipeds) from orthographic images of boxes. As pointed out earlier, when the retinal image is produced by a rectangular box, the observer perceives a rectangular box (a box that has multiple symmetries). This suggested to Perkins that the visual system imposes constraints such as rectangularity when interpreting retinal images. His main question was whether the rectangularity constraint is imposed on the 3D interpretation *only* when the retinal image, and the rules of perspective projection, allow for such an interpretation. In other words, would the observer perceive a rectangular box even when a rectangular box could *not* produce a perspective image equivalent to the retinal image given? Gestalt psychologists claimed that the percept is *only* as good as the prevailing conditions allow (in this case, the shape of the 2D retinal image). This claim suggested that when the rectangular interpretation is not consistent with the retinal image, it will not look like a rectangular box. Perkins' experiment corroborated this suggestion. Specifically, Perkins showed that human observers reliably identified rectangular and nonrectangular parallelepipeds from their orthographic images. This experiment showed two things. First, it showed that the human visual system does use constraints in 3D shape perception. This result was not new. Second, it showed that the visual system "knows" the rules of perspective projection. This result was anticipated by Kaiser (1967) in his experiment with trapezoids, but Kaiser did not point this out because he was more interested in the correlation between shape and slant judgments than in verifying whether the human visual system is a "natural geometer."

Now consider the criterion that the visual system could have used to solve Perkins' task. By using this criterion, the visual system can "decide" whether a rectangular interpretation is possible before the actual 3D shape reconstruction is performed. If a rectangular interpretation is not possible for a given 2D shape on the retina, the rectangularity constraint does not have to be used. In other words, the visual system might "choose" which constraints will be applied depending on the content of the retinal image. Assume that an image of a cube is formed according to an orthographic projection (see figure 2.4). As pointed out above, when the line connecting the center of projection with the vertex of the Y junction of the cube is orthogonal to the image plane, the transformation of the angles at the vertex is the same under orthographic and perspective projection. Therefore, equations derived for an orthographic projection will generalize to a perspective projection. Perkins stated that if the trihedral angle is a right (90 deg) angle, all three angles in the image are obtuse (except for degenerate cases when one or two angles are exactly 90 deg—see figure 2.5a). Perkins did not provide a derivation of this rule, but the derivation is useful for the reader, because only then can the reader see the generality of the final formula or criterion (see appendix B.1). With three edges emanating from a common vertex of a right trihedral angle, either all three have the same direction (away from or toward the observer) or two of them have the same direction. It follows that in the image of a right trihedral angle, either all three angles are obtuse or one is obtuse and two are acute. The line drawing in figure 2.4 satisfies this criterion, but the line drawing in figure 2.5b does not. The reader will probably agree that figure 2.4, but not 2.5b, looks like a rectangular box. The rule derived in appendix B.1 is a somewhat more general version of Perkins' rule. It applies to any junction

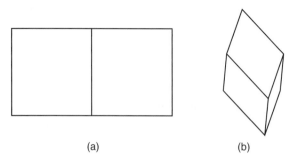

(a)   (b)

Figure 2.5
Applications of Perkins' law: (a) Degenerate case where two angles are equal to 90 deg. (b) An orthographic image of a nonrectangular parallelepiped. This parallelepiped has been obtained by stretching a cube along a diagonal of the base by a factor of three.

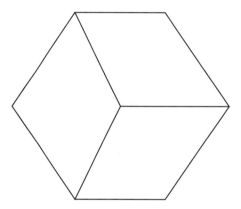

Figure 2.6
An orthographic image of a nonparallelepiped. Note that Perkins's rule is satisfied, but the percept does not correspond to a rectangular parallelepiped, and not even to a parallelepiped.

of three edges in the orthographic image of a cube. The original Perkins' rule was restricted to the Y junction in the center of figure 2.4.

Perkins' rule allows discriminating between images of rectangular and nonrectangular boxes only when the boxes are parallelepipeds (i.e., they have three pairs of parallel faces). If a box is not a parallelepiped, then Perkins' rule is not sufficient. Consider figure 2.6. This box does not look like a rectangular box, and indeed, it is not an image of a rectangular box under orthographic (or perspective) projection even though, according to

Perkins' rule, this box would be classified as rectangular.[5] This means that Perkins' rule itself cannot account for the perceptual classification of images of rectangular versus nonrectangular boxes. This rule must be supplemented with a criterion as to whether the given image could be a projection of a parallelepiped. If we assume that an orthographic projection was used, then the images of edges that are parallel in the 3D space must be parallel in the image. It follows that an orthographic image of a parallelepiped must have three sets of parallel edges. Figure 2.6 violates this criterion. An explanation of how this rule generalizes to a perspective image is given in appendix B (section B.2).

To summarize, the fact that a subject perceives a rectangular box when the retinal image could have been produced by a rectangular box, but does not perceive a rectangular box when it could not have been produced by a rectangular box, implies that the visual system

(i) applies a rectangularity constraint (or some other, similar constraint, like the minimum variance of angles or maximal compactness of the object),

(ii) knows the rules of perspective projection, and

(iii) knows the geometry of its eyeball.

Perkins' results provided support for the first conclusion and partial support for the second. More exactly, Perkins showed that the human visual system knows the rules of orthographic projection. The more general statement about perspective projection follows from examples presented above, and it has been tested experimentally in other studies (e.g., Kaiser, 1967).

Perkins suggested that the rectangularity constraint is similar to the Gestalt psychologists' simplicity principle. This puts Perkins in the neo-Gestaltists' rather than in the Transactionalists' camp; Transactionalists emphasized the role of experience and of visual–motor coordination. They were not nativists (see below).

A natural question arises as to whether the perceptual mechanism involved in viewing pictures (specifically, discriminating between rectangular and nonrectangular boxes in pictures) is different from the mechanism used when actual 3D scenes are viewed. Hochberg and Brooks' (1962) study with a young child suggested that there is one common mechanism. A similar conclusion follows from Perkins and Cooper's (1980) study with groups of children whose mean age was 3, 4.5, and 6 years. These three groups were tested in the task Perkins (1972) had used with adults. Even the youngest group of children could do this task, and their performance was similar to the performance of the college students tested by Perkins (1972). No important differences in performance were observed across the age groups. Perkins and Cooper's evidence provides strong support for the conjecture that the perception of 3D objects from 2D pictures involves the same perceptual mechanism as the perception of the objects themselves.

2.3.2 Reconstruction of Novel Shapes

In his next study, Perkins (1976) generalized the results from his initial study (Perkins, 1972). He examined subjects' ability to reconstruct the shape of an unfamiliar (novel) polyhedron from a single orthographic picture. According to Perkins, if constraints are to be useful in everyday life, they must be a priori, rather than learned, because this would make them applicable to a wide range of objects, including completely novel objects. In this new study, Perkins anticipated modern research on 3D shape perception by (i) emphasizing the role of a priori constraints in 3D shape perception and (ii) showing that constraints alone, without the contribution of depth cues, may be sufficient for veridical 3D shape percept.

The pictures of the polyhedra that were used by Perkins allowed the application of rectangularity, symmetry, and planarity constraints. In fact, when a rectangularity constraint was applied to one of the trihedral angles of a polyhedron (in addition to the planarity constraint being applied to all faces the polyhedron), the shape of the entire polyhedron was specified uniquely. In his previous experiments, Perkins had already demonstrated that subjects apply a rectangularity constraint when the rectangular interpretation is consistent with the retinal image. The new study examined whether subjects perceptually reconstruct the shape of the polyhedron based on the retinal image and the rectangularity constraint. If they do, they should be able to make accurate judgments about this shape. This study was similar to Attneave and Frost's (1969). The main difference is that Attneave and Frost tested the role of regularities (simplicity) in the perception of slant from shape, whereas Perkins (1976) tested the role of regularities in the perception of shape itself.

Subjects were presented with an image of a polyhedron and were asked to estimate the sizes of two angles of the perceived polyhedron. In general, three "regular" interpretations were possible: (i) The first of the two angles was right (90°), (ii) the second angle was right, or (iii) both angles were equal (the object was symmetrical). For some images, only one or even none of the regular interpretations were possible. Eight subjects were tested. Each subject was shown pictures of seven polyhedra. Each picture was shown in eight different orientations.

As in Perkins' previous experiments, the subjects' judgments reflected a systematic application of rectangularity and symmetry constraints to the perceptual interpretation. Furthermore, after the constraint was applied to the perceptual interpretation of one of the angles, the subject judged the other angle accurately. That is, the perceived angle was equal (on average) to the angle in a polyhedron reconstructed from the subject's retinal image by applying planarity, symmetry, and rectangularity constraints. These results provide strong support for Perkins' suggestion that the constraint of rectangularity and symmetry were the kind of Gestalt-like regularities that operate in visual perception. Perkins, however, went beyond the traditional Gestalt thinking. Gestalt psychologists "justified" the use of the simplicity principle by invoking a physiological "cause" in the form of electrical brain currents. Perkins adopted the functional attitude more characteristic of a cognitive psychologist. He claimed that the visual system uses constraints because they allow achieving a veridical percept. He believed that this was true in everyday life, as well as in the case of the impoverished viewing conditions he used in his laboratory. Perkins himself, however, did not provide any experimental evidence for this claim. He never examined realistic viewing conditions in which effective depth cues were available. It would take more than twenty years before such experiments were performed (Pizlo & Stevenson, 1999; Pizlo, Li, & Chan, 2005; Chan et al., 2006).

It is worth pointing out a particularly important implication of Perkins' results. It has been shown in psychophysical experiments that the slant of a plane and the slant of an edge are systematically underestimated regardless of how many effective depth cues are given to the subject (Attneave & Frost, 1969; Perrone, 1980, 1982). However, at the same time, subjects have the ability to interpret images of rectangular boxes as rectangular boxes (Perkins, 1972) and to judge angles of polyhedra accurately (Perkins,

1976). These results clearly imply that *shape is not perceived by taking slant into account*, as many students of perception claimed. If slants of edges and faces were taken into account, a rectangular box would not look rectangular and the angles of a polyhedron would have been systematically misjudged. Neither outcome has ever been reported. This is yet another line of evidence against the Associationists' (or Marr's) explanation of shape perception. *The percept of a 3D shape is not built from elements, that is, piecewise percepts of slants of edges and faces.* It is much more likely that the slants of edges and faces are perceptually derived from the percept of shape, as well as from other cues. Recall that we reached an identical conclusion from Stavrianos' (1945) results, as well as from Attneave and Frost's (1969) results.

2.4   Wallach's Kinetic Depth Effect Reflects a Shift from Nativism to Empiricism

Wallach was included in this section on the contribution of the neo-Gestalt researchers because he received his doctoral training with Köhler, one of the three founding fathers of Gestalt psychology. His research interests after 1950, however, were not directed toward illustrating the role of a simplicity principle in visual perception. He concentrated on the role of (i) higher order stimulus variables, (ii) depth cues, and (iii) past experience in determining the percept. Thus, Wallach's later research represented a shift away from the Gestalt tradition toward a modern version of empiricism. Wallach was especially interested in designing new types of experiments and exploring new phenomena, interests that would challenge existing theories of perceptual mechanisms. Wallach never formulated a general theory of perception, but the collection of his published papers on a broad variety of topics was impressive enough to warrant their publication in book form (Wallach, 1976). Below, I will confine discussion to his papers on the kinetic depth effect (KDE; Wallach & O'Connell, 1953; Wallach et al., 1953) because these are particularly relevant to Wallach's empiristic approach to shape perception. This work stimulated considerable research in computational vision (e.g., Ullman, 1979; Hildreth, 1984). Wallach and O'Connell (1953) begin by making the following claim:

Unfortunately, it appears that no one has succeeded in formulating rules of spontaneous organization adequate to predict which pattern of retinal stimulation will lead to perceived flat figures and which one will produce three-dimensional forms. We have made a vain attempt of our own and have become convinced that the three-dimensional forms perceived in perspective drawings, photographs, etc. are indeed in a matter of previous experience. (pp. 205–6)

By referring to "rules of spontaneous organization," the authors meant the operation of the Gestalt simplicity principle. Their statement is a clear rejection of the simplicity principle as a plausible perceptual mechanism for shape. We now know that simplicity is involved at least in perception of structured solid shapes. This means that Wallach and O'Connell's study was based on an inappropriate assumption. Despite this error, they made an important contribution to our knowledge of depth and shape perception by discovering what they called the KDE. They showed that in the absence of other cues, motion can lead to the three-dimensional percept of an object. Their major claim, however, that the percept of this 3D shape is determined primarily, or even exclusively, by past experience, seems to be false.

Consider now details of the experiments presented in their two papers. In order to eliminate all depth cues other than motion, the subject viewed the shadow of an object rather than the object itself. The object was placed behind a rear-projection screen. Clearly, conventional cues such as binocular disparity, vergence, and accommodation could not provide an observer with any useful information about the shape of the object. If anything, the cues available provided their observers with information suggesting that the distal stimulus was 2D rather than 3D. In the first experiment, they used a solid (opaque) object, so only the occluding contours (outside edges) of the object were visible on the screen. The shadow of a *stationary* solid 3D object does not look like an object. It looks like a 2D figure. However, when the object rotates around an axis orthogonal to the line of sight, its moving shadow leads to the percept of the 3D object. Wallach and O'Connell called this phenomenon the KDE.

The authors did not present any theory of the KDE. That is, they did not explain how the visual system achieves the 3D percept from the motion of a changing 2D shadow on the retina. The first explanation of the KDE was presented by Ullman (1979). Ullman showed that under quite general assumptions, the motion on the retina determines at most one solution equivalent to a rotating rigid object.[6] Ullman's theory can account for most of the results reported by Wallach and O'Connell.

In their second experiment, Wallach and O'Connell (1953) used two wire objects. Their motivation for using wire objects was as follows. In everyday life, a given contour of an object is visible from a wide range of viewing directions. However, when the shadow of an object is presented to the observer, a given contour is perceived only for a narrow range of viewing directions, namely, when this contour happens to be an occluding contour. Using wire objects eliminated this problem, which meant that the wire objects approximated more closely viewing conditions in everyday life than did the solid objects used in their first experiment. The first wire object was a parallelogram containing one diagonal. The parallelogram was bent along this diagonal so that the two parts (triangles) formed an angle of 110 deg. The second wire object was a helix. It was a polygonal line consisting of three straight-line segments. When the object was stationary, the shadow led to a 2D rather than 3D percept. When the object rotated, the observer was likely to see a 3D object. Each subject was shown one of the objects rotating for 10 seconds. Presentations were repeated until the subject produced a "clear report." Most of the fifty subjects tested achieved the 3D percept, sooner or later. For sixteen of the subjects, the authors recorded whether they achieved the 3D percept after the first 10-second presentation. Eleven reported a 3D percept with the "parallelogram," but only four reported a 3D percept with the helix. The low rate of subjects' reporting 3D percepts with the helix suggests that the visual system has difficulty reconstructing the object from a moving shadow when the object is unstructured.[7]

In the next several experiments, Wallach and his coworkers studied the robustness of the KDE and reported that when the shadow expands and contracts in only one direction, the KDE is absent. Such conditions are present when a rectangle rotates around one of its sides, and this side is orthogonal to the line of sight. When the visible contours of the object are curved and do not have distinctive points, the KDE is weak or absent altogether. Finally, when only angles, but not distances, change in the shadow, the KDE is absent again. Such conditions are present when the shadow of a Y junction forming a trihedral angle is shown through an aperture in such a way that the endpoints are not visible. Once again, the authors did not provide any explanation of these failures to produce the KDE. One possible explanation is based on the fact that in these cases, the information available on the retina is simply not sufficient for a unique reconstruction (Ullman, 1979). Next, Wallach and O'Connell (1953) showed that stimuli that do not ordinarily produce the KDE may be able to produce the KDE if the presentation of the initially ineffective stimulus is preceded by another stimulus, a stimulus that produces a reliable KDE.

The last experiment of interest in Wallach and O'Connell's (1953) study was a test of the veridicality of the percept produced by moving shadows of the bent wire parallelogram used in their second experiment. Subjects were asked to identify the wire shape that had produced the moving shadow. Four comparison parallelograms were used with the angle between the two planar parts being equal to 95, 110, 125, and 140 deg (the test parallelogram had an angle of 110 deg). Thirty subjects were tested with the four comparison stimuli. More than half of their choices were correct. These results indicate that the KDE can produce a rather reliable perception of shape.

Wallach, O'Connell, and Neisser (1953) went on to examine the role memory might play in establishing a 3D percept. The three stimuli and procedure used in Wallach and O'Connell's (1953) study were used in this study. The authors first demonstrated that the frequency with which the subject saw the shadow as a 3D object, when the object was stationary, was substantially increased if the stationary presentation was preceded by a moving exposure of this object. The authors then showed that this result does not generalize across objects: A moving exposure of one object *does not* increase the frequency of seeing another object as 3D when it was tested with a stationary presentation. These results show clearly that when there is perceptual learning of 3D shapes, learning is not taking place at the level of the perceptual mechanisms. Learning is limited to memorizing the shapes of individual objects. Wallach et al. (1953) claimed that the KDE is fundamental, providing a monocular mechanism for learning to perceive 3D shapes as one moves about in the environment. However, more recent studies by Slater and Morrison (1985) on the perception of shapes in newborn infants suggest otherwise.

To summarize, perception of 3D shape involves a one-to-many mapping between the retina and the percept: This mapping represents the reconstruction of the third dimension (depth). Therefore, any theory of 3D shape perception must explain how the 3D rather than the 2D interpretation is produced from a 2D image. Reconstructing a 3D shape from a 2D image cannot rely exclusively on *removing* redundancy from the image, a concern of many over many years (e.g., "stripping the sensory messages of their redundancy," Attneave, 1954, p. 189; Barlow, 1961, p. 223; "squeezing out regularities," van der Helm, 2000, p. 787). It is clear that reconstructing 3D shape from its 2D image must rely on *adding* information to the 2D image, not on simplifying it!

In short, *we perceive the 3D world as 3D, rather than as 2D, not because the 3D interpretation is simpler, which it may very well be, at least on some occasions, but because it is a smart thing to do.* This claim spells out the main difference between the Gestalt and the cognitive approach to perception.

2.5   Empiricism Revisited

Progress in understanding shape perception achieved during the first half of the twentieth century, which was stimulated almost exclusively by the Gestalt psychologists, was based on introducing the concept of a priori rules of perceptual organization. The Gestalt psychologists not only introduced these a priori rules into the study of perception but also provided many powerful illustrations of how these rules impose constraints on the family of possible perceptual interpretations. The Cognitive Revolution during the 1950s and 1960s contributed to understanding shape perception by showing that the Gestalt rules of perceptual organization could, in principle, be formulated in the language of information theory in ways that might even play a critical role in achieving veridical percepts. The work done in this period, however, was not based on formalisms included in information theory, so understanding shape did not progress very far, and in fact, it is not entirely clear that even if researchers had tried these formalisms, they would have succeeded (Luce, 2003). The line of research based on the concept of a simplicity principle was interrupted for a couple of decades by attempts to revive the empiristic approach to shape perception, the approach that was started by Locke, developed by Berkeley, and championed at the beginning of the modern era by Helmholtz.

Empiricism in this period added some novel elements. First, neuroscience became a prominent component of cognitive psychology, encouraging the development of neural network models. Second, the Gestalt psychologists' emphasis upon automatic, a priori perceptual processing left little or no room for the influence of high-level processes such as memory, learning, motivation, and social interaction. Psychologists interested in a role for higher processes in perception felt neglected and sought to introduce a "New Look" into the study of perception, including shape. The development of neural neo-empiricism was led by Hebb (1949). The New Look in perception was led by Bruner and Goodman (1947).

Hebb (1949), in a widely cited book, proposed an empiristic, neurally based, motor-learning theory of 2D shape perception as an alternative to the nativistic theory of the Gestalt psychologists. He realized that trying to revive empiricism in the period following the success of Gestalt psychology required assuming at least one innate perceptual accomplishment on the basis of which the organism could learn to perceive shapes. He called this innate perceptual accomplishment "primitive unity." Primitive unity corresponded to the percept of a discriminable region whose brightness was different from the rest of the visual field (a smudge). This smudge was functionally analogous to the figure–ground organization of the Gestalt psychologists, except for a critical difference, namely, Hebb's primitive unity did not have a contour and thus had no shape. Prolonged and repeated fixations on discontinuities produced by edges and corners in the visual field led to the formation of brain circuits Hebb called "cell-assemblies." These were the physiological correlates of the perception of edges and corners. Once these perceptual elements were established, they were integrated to produce a percept of shape. The percept of shape, as well as the presence of edges and corners, was learned. Shapes were learned by making repetitive eye movements along the contours. Specifically, the percept of a 2D shape resulted from learning sequences of (i) percepts of corners of figures and (ii) eye movements that took the line of sight from one corner to another. On the physiological level, learning was assumed to involve changing the strength of synaptic connections among neurons. After a sequence of percepts and eye movements (called a "phase sequence") is established, the percept of shape can be produced without actually moving the eye, but merely by being ready to do so. Hebb is often given credit for the first formulation of "connectionism," a branch of computational neuroscience popular during the last twenty years (Rumelhart & McClelland, 1986). His emphasis on learning at the neural level had a lasting impact. It is now referred to as the "Hebbian learning rule." The perceptual–motor part of his theory of shape did not survive.[8]

Bruner and Goodman (1947), reacting to a different aspect of the success of Gestalt psychology, introduced what they called the "New Look" approach to perception. The Gestalt psychologists emphasized what we would now call the "bottom-up" aspects of perceptual processing. The observer is passive; his or her innate organizing processes automatically impose structure on the retinal image of the visual world. The observer's personal characteristics did not enter into the information received. The New Lookers, on the other hand, emphasized "top-down" processing: the role of an individual's needs, values, and expectations in the way the retinal image would be processed by the brain. Bruner described this as "going beyond the information given" (Bruner, 1957; Bruner, Goodnow, & Austin, 1956). The support for the New Look was obtained in experiments demonstrating what has been called "perceptual defense," in which tachistoscopic presentations of taboo words produced longer response times than presentation of ordinary words. Bruner also demonstrated what he believed to be a role of personal values in size perception, supporting this claim with experiments that showed that poor children overestimated the size of a quarter, whereas rich children did not. Bruner also claimed that the perceived shapes of simple ambiguous drawings reflected the needs of the subjects. He supported this by showing that hungry subjects described seeing more food objects than did subjects who were not hungry. This kind of research produced a flurry of activity for a decade. All of these effects were ultimately shown to be artifacts. They could be explained by simpler mechanisms, namely, "response availability" and "response suppression." Simply put, everyone perceives these ambiguous stimuli the same way but describes them differently, depending on their backgrounds, needs, and expectations.

There was another development in this neo-empiristic period, which also failed to produce lasting effects. It called attention to the role of past experience, primarily in size and depth perception. This approach was taken by the Transactionalists, who were led by Adalbert Ames, Jr. The concept of "transaction" was introduced to convey the idea that perception cannot be analyzed in isolation, independent of the prior experience of the observer, of his or her current goals, as well as of the consequences of actions taken to achieve these goals, such as looking around, bringing an object nearer, changing its orientation, and so forth. Ames, the founder of the Transactional School, started his school by introducing, in the late 1930s, powerful demonstrations illustrating the role of familiarity in determining what is perceived (Cantril, 1960). One of the best known involved a set of unconnected rods and a parallelogram, arranged in such a way that from one viewing direction these elements produced an image of a chair in the observer's eye. From this, and only from this, viewing direction, a monocular observer saw a chair, rather than the actual haphazard 3D arrangement of parts of a chair (figure 2.7—after Kilpatrick, 1961, p. 38). The Transactionalists' explanation of this phenomenon says that when we look at real chairs, tables, boxes, and rooms, we perceive them as rectangular, even though nonrectangular interpretations are possible, because in the past, we had seen only rectangular chairs, tables, boxes, and rooms. In other words, we know that rectangular objects are likely to be encountered in our environment, and this is what we see whenever such interpretations are consistent with the retinal image. Clearly, the Transactionalists attributed to experience and a likelihood principle what the Gestalt psychologists attributed to innate rules involving a simplicity principle. Transactionalists made numerous attempts to demonstrate the role of learning in shape perception, by using distorted objects and rooms, but they provided very limited, if any, evidence for this position. Their experiments were analogous to those of Stratton (1896) and Ivo Kohler (1962), who introduced distortions by having subjects view the world through prisms or inverting goggles. All these experiments showed that subjects can learn how to behave in the presence of a distorted environment, but they did not come to confuse them with normal environments even after they learned to perform quite

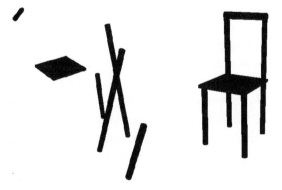

Figure 2.7
Ames chair demonstration (after Kilpatrick, 1961). These images were produced using 3D graphics software (3DS Max/Autodesk) rather than physical materials.

complicated visually guided behaviors within them (Linden et al., 1999). Significant learning effects on perception seem to be limited to depth, size, and direction. Perception of shape has never been shown to be affected by learning.

The role of learning in perception was also championed by Rock (1977, 1983), who is often classified as an empiricist. Rock's work is important because he is credited for reviving Helmhotz' (1910) concept of unconscious inference in perception. Rock popularized the notion of unconscious inference, ascribing it to Helmholtz, but, whereas Helmholtz assumed that the visual system memorizes individual objects and then uses these memories in subsequent perceptions, Rock assumed that the visual system is "smart" and uses rules of geometrical optics and principles of logic as well as probability calculus. This shift of emphasis from associative learning to unconscious thinking is illustrated by the title of Rock's (1983) book: *The Logic of Perception.*[9]

Rock, unlike Helmholtz, downplayed the importance of associative learning and emphasized cognitive processes. This is not surprising because during his education and early career he was influenced by Gestalt psychologists. His doctoral mentor was Hans Wallach. However, as he continued to develop his perception models, he found it necessary to use simple learning models along with more cognitive mechanisms (Rock, 1983). It seems that Rock's shift toward empiricism was stimulated by his emphasis on the veridicality of the percept. He did not see why an intelligent system should try to emphasize the simplicity of perceptual representation when the task is actually to produce veridical percepts (Rock, 1983, p. 164). It is easy to see that simplicity might be an innate principle, whereas the bias toward veridicality is more likely to be related to our experiences and interactions within the environment. By shifting from a Gestalt way of thinking to a Helmholtzian way of thinking, Rock lost the benefits inherent in the Gestalt concept of perceptual organization. Once he made this shift, he thought that the accuracy of a percept depended more on visual cues than on perceptual organization once both experience and learning played an important role in perception. What was obvious to Gestalt psychologists, as well as to Transactional psychologists, was not obvious to Rock. His assumption that perceptual organization is not needed made Rock's theory similar to Gibson's, although Gibson did not think that visual perception involved any computation or reasoning as Rock did.

Clearly, Rock's theory represents an unusual combination of elements taken from several, often conflicting approaches.

Rock's interest in shape started with 2D shapes (Rock, 1973, 1983). We already knew that the perception of the shapes of 2D line drawings, such as a square, does not involve simplicity constraints (see chapter 1). Therefore, it is not surprising that Rock did not see any use for a simplicity principle in the case of 2D shapes. In his table 1–1 (Rock, 1983, p. 18), Rock states that perceiving the shape of an object is tantamount to describing its shape. No reconstruction is needed. For example, a square and a diamond are perceptually different only in where the "top" is assigned. This difference does not require invoking any simplicity principle. After characterizing the perception of 2D shape as a process of description, Rock moved on to the case of 3D shapes and stated, without much justification, the following:

What has been said about two dimensions can easily be extended to the third. Thus it seems probable that few if any entirely new principles need be invoked to deal with object-form perception in daily life. Presumably the shape of each face of an object is described as a two-dimensional structure and depth relations are incorporated into the overall description insofar as they yield spatial relationships about the structure of the object. (p. 87)

The reader will soon see that despite large differences between their theoretical positions, both Rock and Gibson fell victim to the same problem: They underestimated the inherent computational difficulty of reconstructing 3D spatial relations. Gibson claimed that we see 3D space directly, and Rock claimed that the observer's task was simply to describe 3D space. Neither of them actually tried to verify these claims in computer simulations. Had they done so, they would have undoubtedly realized that constraints are critical.

To test his ideas about the perception of 3D shapes, Rock performed a sequence of experiments using unstructured wire objects like the one shown in figure 2.8 (Rock, DiVita, & Barbeito, 1981; Rock & DiVita, 1987; Rock, Wheeler, & Tudor, 1989). These experiments stimulated others to study 3D shape perception. These wire objects were viewed binocularly from a distance between 0.5 and 1.25 m (different viewing distances were used in different studies). The subject was shown an object from two different viewing directions (45 or 90 deg apart) and was asked to recognize the object based on its shape. This was, in effect, a shape constancy

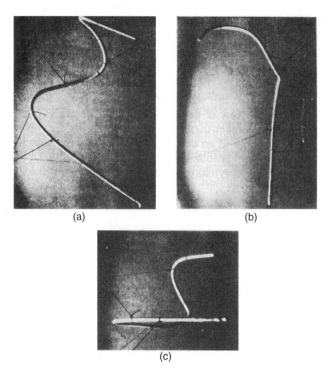

(a)   (b)

(c)

Figure 2.8
Three views of a wire object used by Rock, DiVita, and Barbeito (1981, from Rock, 1983, p. 88—with kind permission of Sylvia Rock).

experiment, using unfamiliar, meaningless, unstructured objects. The main reason Rock used wire objects was to avoid self-occlusion. With ordinary opaque objects, we can see only one half of the object's surface. Rock expected that binocular viewing from a fairly close distance would allow the subject to use depth cues to perceive the wire object's entire 3D shape. Rock assumed that the simplicity principle is not important in 3D shape perception, so from his point of view the simplicity of his stimuli should not matter. The design of Rock's experiments was obviously based on his theoretical approach.

The main result of Rock's three studies with wire figures was that shape constancy failed completely! Unfamiliar, unstructured 3D wire objects, rotated in depth by 45–90 deg, could not be recognized as the same object viewed from a different viewpoint. Rock wrote as follows: "Since the figures are seen under conditions of adequate depth information, there is no difficulty in recovering the internal spatial relations that characterize the object's shape. Bearing in mind that no part of the figure is hidden, the shape should be described in the same way regardless of the observer's vantage point" (Rock, 1983, p. 88). The fact that the percept was dramatically affected by changing the observer's vantage point encouraged Rock to conclude that 3D shapes are only represented perceptually in the viewer-centered coordinate system. The viewer-centered description of an object involves depths and orientations of edges and surfaces relative to the observer, but not relational properties characterizing shape. As you will see, Rock's thinking seems to have been influenced by Marr's 2.5D sketch (see chapter 3 for Marr's theory). If it was, considering the wide differences in their backgrounds and training, Marr had clearly captured the zeitgeist of the period.

In 1989, Rock began to have some doubts about whether his subjects had been able to perceive the wire objects in depth veridically. They had to be able to do this in order to form a viewer-centered 3D description of the objects. This concern led to a new experiment with his 3D wire objects in which depth perception was tested directly (Rock et al., 1989). In one condition, subjects were asked to judge the ratio of width to depth and the ratio of height to depth of his 3D wire objects. Rock et al. (1989) found that the aspect ratios (averaged across eight subjects) were very close to the actual aspect ratios, encouraging them to conclude that depth had been perceived veridically. From Rock's point of view, this meant that the failure to demonstrate shape constancy could not be attributed to an unreliable perception of depth or to the inability to form a viewer-centered representation of the 3D wire objects. This led Rock et al. to conclude that the human visual system does not form an object-centered representation of shapes (pp. 203–204). In other words, we don't perceive 3D shapes as shapes, but only as a collection of surface orientations and depths. Note, however, that it is more likely that the real reason Rock et al. failed to obtain shape constancy was their use of very unnatural, unstructured stimuli. The shape of such wire objects is not well specified because they do not have sufficient surfaces and volume. In effect, the shape of such objects does not fall within the large class of objects where simplicity constraints can operate. We will see later why these constraints are essential for the veridical perception of 3D shapes, that is, for achieving shape constancy.

We see in Rock's work another example of how the willingness to use "taking into account" explanations for the perception of shape can lead one astray. Both Rock and Thouless studied variables (depth and 3D orientation) that they believed were directly related to shape constancy through a "taking into account" explanation. They did not study shape itself. Thouless used ellipses. This was a problem because an ellipse is not sufficiently complex—its shape is characterized by only one parameter that can be arbitrarily changed in the perspective projection to the retina. As a result, the retinal images of his ellipses did not provide enough information, and shape constancy failed. Rock used unstructured 3D wire objects. This was a problem because there is no definition of "simplicity" that, when applied to the retinal image of such a 3D wire object, could allow the reconstruction of a unique 3D object. Note that *shape constancy depends critically on the operation of a simplicity principle, and the shape perceived cannot be constant (the same) unless the percept is unique.* The retinal image of a 3D wire object simply does not provide enough information for the percept to be unique, so shape constancy failed with Rock's wire objects just as it did with Thouless' ellipses.

To summarize, the main conceptual contribution of neo-empiricism was the reformulation of Helmholtzian empiricism in the language of cognitive psychology. Once this was done, the visual system no longer solved constancy problems by using "look-up tables" as claimed by Berkeley and Helmholtz. Instead, constancy problems are solved actively by logical processing. Adopting this approach makes the modern view very similar to Descartes' except in one respect. According to Descartes, the human observer was a "natural geometer," whose knowledge of geometry was innate. According to the neo-empiricists, the human observer must learn the rules of geometry. So far, contemporary neo-empiricists have not provided evidence to demonstrate that the rules are learned. They did, however, contribute by emphasizing the importance of (i) studying the perception of the shapes of 3D objects and (ii) veridicality in shape perception. Both of these contributions will figure prominently in the development of machine vision.

There were other, somewhat tangential, developments during this period. Particularly notable was one introduced by Gregory (1968), who provided a particularly striking example to illustrate the difficulties facing traditional explanations of the cognitive psychologists, who were looking for a universal rule that could explain the percept of a 3D object from the object's retinal image. Neo-Gestaltists, such as Hochberg and McAlister (1953) and Leeuwenberg (1971), were trying to formulate a simplicity principle using the formalism of information theory, whereas neo-empiricists were trying to formulate a likelihood principle using probability theory (e.g., Brunswik, 1956; Kilpatrick, 1961; Rock, 1983). Gregory provided a challenge to these two approaches that suggested that neither was likely to succeed. He used Penrose and Penrose's (1958) "impossible triangle" shown in figure 2.9. This looks like a 3D object, but clearly a physical object that actually looked like this could not be constructed. If this is not obvious, look closely at the individual corners of this "triangular object." It is clear that the perceptual interpretation of any two corners of this triangle is inconsistent with the interpretation of the third. Note, however, that the fact we see an "impossible object" in figure 2.9 does not prove that there is no physical object that could actually produce a picture like this. Gregory (1968) showed that there is such a physical object. It is shown in figure 2.10. Why is Gregory's object a problem? The percept of an impossible object is a problem for the neo-empiristic explanation because we see an object that we have never seen before. How can an impossible 3D object be more likely than a possible object? This "impossible" percept also pres-

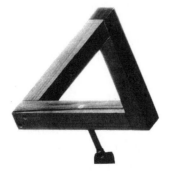

Figure 2.9
This figure, taken from Gregory (*The intelligent eye*, 1970, with permission of The McGraw-Hill companies and of the author), shows an object with a triangular shape. However, on close examination, it is clear that a physical object like this could not actually be assembled. Each of the three corners look three-dimensional, but the three corners shown in this figure cannot form a 3D object like this.

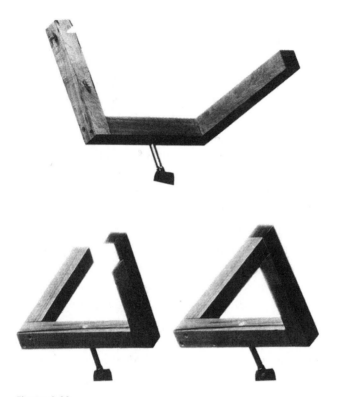

Figure 2.10
Three views taken from different viewing directions of the object shown in figure 2.9. Here, it can be seen on the bottom right. Gregory used this figure to illustrate that Penrose and Penrose's (1958) object could actually be assembled but it did not have a closed triangular shape when viewed from the viewpoint illustrated on the bottom right (from Gregory, *The intelligent eye*, 1970, with permission of The McGraw-Hill companies and of the author).

ents a problem for the neo-Gestalt approach because no definition of simplicity is available according to which an impossible 3D interpretation is simpler than a possible interpretation, and simpler than its 2D image, itself. Gregory's demonstration suggests that neither a simplicity nor a likelihood principle can predict what would be seen. Either principle will have to be modified to deal with individual parts of the image separately (Hochberg, 1978). Furthermore, these operations most surely will have to be preceded by some operation that establishes that the object is a "closed" triangle, which, in itself, requires the operation of a simplicity or likelihood

principle. Thus, individuals working within either the nativistic or empiristic tradition were faced with the task of formulating a computational
model of the underlying perceptual mechanisms. Explaining perceived
shape cannot be done simply by providing a definition of simplicity.
Instead, one has to specify the computations and the order in which they
should be performed. Both of these issues will figure prominently in the
development of machine vision.

3   Machine Vision

As we have just seen, simply trying to refine and perfect definitions of simplicity will not make it possible to explain how shape constancy is achieved. The goal (or purpose) of shape constancy is not to produce simple percepts, as the Gestalt psychologists and those they influenced proposed, because constancy is needed and achieved with quite complex shapes. Ecologically significant shapes are by no means always simple. The goal (or purpose) of shape constancy, as Perkins and those he influenced proposed, was to produce veridical percepts. Once this is appreciated, it is clear that a useful definition of "simplicity" in the case of shape should be based on testing computational models of shape constancy. By the 1970s the formulation of such models was being attempted both by psychologists who were trying to understand biological vision systems and by engineers who were trying to design machines with visual abilities. Only the contributions of the machine vision community will be discussed in this chapter.[1]

Selfridge and Neisser (1960), a computer scientist and a psychologist, respectively, were among the first to tackle a machine vision problem, namely, character recognition. Solving this problem would have practical implications. It would allow machines to process checks. Selfridge and Neisser showed that it is possible to program a computer to recognize letters with a familiar font by means of template matching. However, it was almost impossible to do this with an unfamiliar font or with handwriting whose font is idiosyncratic. Recognition was better when features of letters, rather than conventional letters, were used. However, even when computer programs could recognize isolated conventional letters, they could not recognize groups of letters such as words, phrases, and sentences.

In fact, this task, which every human reader does easily, can still not be done well by machines.

Observations in sensory neurophysiology made during the 1950s, specifically lateral inhibition in limulus optic nerve (Hartline & Ratliff, 1957), center-surround organization in the cat's retina (Kuffler, 1953), and Lettvin's specialized feature detectors in the frog's retina (Lettvin et al., 1951), suggested that simple sensory phenomena like these are probably based on simple mechanisms that can be modeled with simple transistor networks (Pitts & McCulloch, 1947; McCulloch & Pitts, 1943; Rosenblatt, 1962). It was hoped that simulation of simple neural circuits, like these, could be scaled up to allow explanation of much more complex perceptual accomplishments such as shape perception and even problem solving. This hope was only partially realized. Namely, it led to computer programs that could recognize very simple properties of 2D patterns, but by 1969, Minsky and Pappert pointed out that this endeavor was fundamentally limited. It cannot be scaled up to the level of 3D shapes because 3D shapes are complex. Shapes, both 3D and 2D, require very many parameters, so no simple feature detector can accomplish the task of shape description or recognition (see the discussion associated with figure 1.1). Minsky and Pappert's (1969) book was extremely influential. It discouraged further development of overly simplistic neural networks for a couple of decades. By the mid-1980s, "neural networks," embellished with new learning mechanisms, such as the "generalized delta rule," made an enthusiastic comeback. This comeback bore the name "parallel distributed processing" (Rumelhart & McClelland, 1986). Unfortunately, progress in this area has not brought us any closer to understanding 3D shape perception as many were convinced it would when it was introduced.

Meanwhile, another group of engineers started working on a set of problems related to the interpretation of 3D scenes and shapes. This work was motivated by robotic applications, such as finding and picking up manufacturing parts and manipulating tools on production lines. This approach is often referred to as "robot vision." It was successful because the variety of objects that had to be found, picked up, and manipulated was restricted. Roberts (1965) pioneered this approach when he developed a matching algorithm for recognizing a 3D shape, represented by a set of points, from its camera (single-perspective) image. This method, however, could only be applied to simple 3D polyhedral objects. Roberts himself tested his algorithm with only three polyhedra: a cube, a wedge, and a hexagonal prism.

Roberts was primarily interested in having a robot recognize a simple 3D object from a set of familiar objects whose models were stored in the robot's database. His main contribution was to address the issue of 3D shapes when others who were interested in machine vision were only dealing with 2D shapes, such as alphanumeric characters. The problem of recognizing a 3D shape from its perspective image is directly related to what is known in the psychological literature as "shape constancy."[2] Recall that "shape constancy" refers to the fact that the percept of the shape of a given object remains the same despite changes in the object's retinal image caused by changes in the viewing direction. Roberts, by using 3D objects, avoided problems inherent in earlier research on shape constancy. Recall, simple 2D shapes, such as ellipses, did not allow Thouless to actually study, much less to solve, the problem of shape constancy. Roberts' contribution was significant because it is not trivial to solve the shape constancy problem in the case of complex 3D shapes. Roberts paved the way for doing this by using projective geometry. Consider the nature of this problem. Perspective projection is a nonlinear transformation (see appendix C, section C.2, for equations defining a 3D to 2D perspective projection). As a result, matching a 3D shape with a 2D image involves nonlinear equations that are difficult to solve analytically. Roberts realized that this problem can be greatly simplified when "homogeneous" rather than Euclidean coordinates are used (appendix C, section C.3).[3] Roberts' (1965) use of linear equations was clever because it allowed him to handle the perspective projection by means of matrix algebra.

One aspect of Roberts' method is worth highlighting. By using homogeneous coordinates, he effectively changed the problem of recognizing 3D shapes as represented by ratios of *Euclidean* distances to the problem of recognizing shapes as represented by their *projective* structure.[4] Figure 3.1 illustrates the difference between *Euclidean* (a) and *projective* (b) structures. Figure 3.1a shows an image of a cube. In this case, the reader will perceive a cube providing the viewing distance is several times larger than the size of the image. In contrast, figure 3.1b shows an image of a 3D projective transformation of a cube. The reader will not perceive this shape as a cube: (a) and (b) are perceived as different shapes. However, for Roberts' algorithm, (a) and (b) are perceived as the same shape. Clearly, Roberts' method

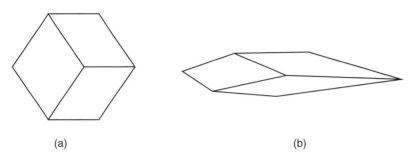

(a)   (b)

Figure 3.1
(a) An image of a cube. When the reader views this image from a large viewing distance, the retinal image is a valid perspective projection of a cube and the viewer perceives a cube, that is, a rectangular box whose edges all have identical lengths. (b) An image of a *projective* transformation of a cube. Projective transformation changes size as well as shape. Here we are only concerned with shape, not size. A projective transformation of a cube does not have right angles, and its edges have different lengths. The human observer does not perceive (b) as a cube. However, when Roberts' method using homogeneous coordinates is applied to these drawings, both (a) and (b) will "look" like cubes, that is, a rectangular box with equal sides (after Pizlo & Scheessele, 1998).

is different from the method used by the human visual system, in the sense that it can "recognize" shapes despite considerable distortions. Humans do not. They see a shape and its projective transformation as very different shapes.

Shortly after Roberts published his seminal work, a series of papers appeared providing methods for machine interpretation of line drawings of objects. Whereas Roberts was interested in identifying and discriminating individual objects, this new work emphasized understanding a complex 3D scene composed of complex objects, such as polyhedra. Note that once we speak of an object in a complex scene, figure–ground organization looms large: One has to identify which of the contours belong to the object and which to the background. From the point of view of a human observer, it is a trivial problem, and the resulting percept is almost always veridical. From the engineering point of view, figure–ground organization is extremely difficult, so it is not surprising that progress was slow.

Guzman (1968) began by describing a method for decomposing an image into regions corresponding to individual objects. He used images of polyhedral objects and showed that the individual objects can be identified despite partial occlusions in the image. This result is quite interesting because it shows that figure–ground organization may be tractable, as long as the "figures" are images of 3D objects. Most, if not all, of the previous research on human figure–ground organization used 2D, "toy" stimuli, rather than realistic images of solid objects. Note that there is a hint here that solving the 3D shape constancy problem may be easier than solving a 2D shape constancy problem—a hint, however, that was not noticed by those who studied the shape constancy problem with simple 2D figures. Clowes (1971) and Huffman (1971) extended Guzman's work by formulating criteria that allowed classifying edges and trihedral vertices of corners into convex and concave. Waltz (1972) added constraints to this classification by using information about shading. In fact, Waltz' method was usually able to produce a unique (and accurate) interpretation of line drawings of polyhedra. It is important to point out that interpretation of a line drawing as representing 3D objects involves solving two related problems. The first is determining which parts of the image represent individual objects and parts of the objects (figure–ground organization), and the second is providing a 3D representation of the objects. The latter cannot be done without the former. In other words, figure–ground organization *must precede* 3D representation.

All these early papers concentrated on qualitative aspects of shape (e.g., deciding between convex and concave corners). As a result, a polyhedron could often be reconstructed, but the sizes of the angles of the polyhedron remained unknown. Recall, however, that Roberts' recognition method did not allow recognizing angles, either, because it involved recognizing projective, not Euclidean, structure. Interestingly, there is a close similarity between the results produced by Roberts' recognition method and the reconstruction of polyhedra from a single image.[5]

Mackworth (1973) and later Kanade (1981) improved the reconstruction methods by adding quantitative constraints that restricted the family of possible polyhedra. For example, if a face of the polyhedron is symmetrical, then the family of possible orientations of the polygon characterized by slant and tilt is represented by only one free parameter (Kanade, 1981). This line of research culminated in Sugihara's (1986) work. Sugihara formulated the necessary and sufficient conditions for a line drawing to represent a physically realizable (possible vs. impossible) polyhedron. Sugihara's work was the starting point for two different lines of research that are directly related to human shape perception. One line of research involved what is called "model-based invariants" for shape recognition, and the other involved what is called "optimization-based reconstruction of shapes." In both, the visual system is assumed to apply some operations to a 2D shape on the retina in order to provide a percept of a 3D shape. It follows that figure–ground organization must be performed first in order to find the 2D shapes on the retina. Clearly, figure–ground organization and shape recognition and reconstruction are two closely related aspects of the perception of 3D objects. This was appreciated, and both were treated as such by researchers of that period. Unfortunately, Sugihara's approach emerged at a time when a major innovator came on the scene, an innovator who took a novel approach to shape perception that pushed Sugihara's approach into the background for many years.

The innovator was David Marr (1982). He was the first to explicitly address the issue of computational modeling of the entire human visual system rather than concentrating on simple, but tractable problems of reconstructing and recognizing simple objects. By turning the attention of both the human and machine vision communities to human vision, Marr, in fact, addressed the "big problem" of formulating a computational theory of a general-purpose vision system. By that he meant a system that can work with real images (as opposed to line drawings) and can be applied to a wide range of objects, not only polyhedra. This emphasis represented breaking with traditional approaches in both human vision and machine vision. Marr was the first to capitalize on the observation that interpreting real images of natural scenes is much harder than interpreting synthetic images of toy scenes. However, once real images, rather than line drawings, are of interest, the computational complexity of the problem requires the use of computers—analytical treatment is usually not possible. Further-more, Marr realized that simulations are particularly important because they dramatically restrict the family of possible theories of human vision. If a computational model does not lead to reliable reconstruction of a 3D visual scene, it cannot be useful as a model of human vision. The human visual system is highly effective, as well as very reliable, when it is used to interpret real images of natural scenes. Marr's formulation of visual percep-tion was revolutionary. It contained so many insightful ideas that his approach was adopted by almost all researchers interested in space and shape perception during the last twenty years of the twentieth century.

Marr's approach was so influential that it is usually referred to as "Marr's paradigm." Marr deserves special credit because he encouraged vision scientists with diverse backgrounds to take an interest in solving the "big problem" he raised, namely, formulating a computational theory for interpreting real images of natural scenes. He, and those he attracted, failed to do this, but their efforts provided new insights into the problem of shape perception that were elaborated by those he influenced. The strengths and weaknesses of Marr's approach will be discussed next.

3.1 Marr's Computational Vision

Marr's paradigm can be best characterized by discussing some of his assumptions: namely,

(i) space and shape perception are the most important issues in vision,

(ii) visual perception involves information processing,

(iii) the perception of 3D shape is based on perception of surface orientation,

(iv) the representation and recognition of 3D shapes involves 3D models, and

(v) it is possible to develop a new theory of human shape perception without concurrent psychophysical experiments to test its plausibility and/ or without making the new theory consistent with existing psychophysical data obtained from human observers.

3.1.1 Space and Shape Perception

Marr began by asking about the purpose of vision. Evidence from patients who suffered localized and specific brain damage suggested to him that shape and space can be reconstructed on the basis of visual information alone. The meaning, familiarity, or importance of the objects contained within the space are not needed (Marr, 1982, pp. 34–46). Here, Marr is reflecting the Zeitgeist in neuroscience, which was emphasizing the "modularity" of brain functions in his day. Neuroscientists were very busy demonstrating that different specialized regions within the brain were responsible for performing different functions. Marr then added the claim that shape and space perception are *the* most important visual properties. Other properties such as color, texture, or motion are secondary (p. 36).

Marr did not justify his claim about the relative importance of shape except for saying that once we understand shape perception, it will be easy to add the other properties. His book, which he titled *Vision*, concentrated almost exclusively on the perception of shape and space.

3.1.2 Visual Perception Involves Information Processing

Marr introduces this discussion by describing the main flaw inherent in Gibson's approach. According to Gibson's approach, called "direct percep-tion," accurate perceptions of space and shape are based on invariants that reside in the environment and can be effortlessly "picked up" by the observer. Specifically, the visual system, according to Gibson, does not have to compute anything in order to produce a veridical representation of 3D shape, as long as the viewer is allowed to use both eyes and to move about freely. Simply put, Gibson was engaged in wishful thinking. He grossly underestimated the difficulty of reconstructing 3D visual space. The source of this difficulty, of course, derives from the well-known fact that the visual system obtains information about the 3D world from 2D representations on the retinas. The retinal image is a perspective transformation of the 3D scene and, therefore, does not allow "direct" measurement of Euclidean properties of the scene such as shape. The visual system *can* use invariants of a perspective transformation, but these invariants (projective) do not uniquely specify a 3D shape, as illustrated in figure 3.1 (see appendix C, section C.1b, for classification of invariants that are relevant to shape per-ception). Both parts of figure 3.1 represent the same shape from the point of view of projective geometry, but these two figures are perceived as having different shapes. Projective invariants can be useful in discriminat-ing very different shapes but cannot be used in reconstructing novel shapes. However, even if invariants are used to discriminate shapes, invari-ants have to be computed, not just "picked up." They are not simply lying around in the environment. To be sure, Gibson deserves credit for insisting that an adequate study of human vision must involve 3D scenes and shapes because in his day, the commonly adopted approach was rooted in Fechnerian psychophysics (Fechner, 1860). In Fechnerian psychophysics, the percept of the natural environment is constructed from simple ele-ments such as sensations of brightness, color, and contrast. Fechner, and all who followed in his tradition, did not even begin to deal with the per-ception of real objects in natural environments. Thus, Gibson's emphasis on the importance of studying perception of 3D scenes was valuable, but his "theory" of 3D perception was not. It was Marr who realized that 3D space and shape perception is a difficult computational problem that *must* be attacked as such.

3.1.3 Perception of 3D Shape Is Based on Perception of Surface Orientation

The perceptual representation of surface orientation and distance relative to the viewer was central in Marr's computational theory of shape. Marr called this representation a 2.5D sketch. The label, "2.5D," rather than 3D, derives from the fact that we usually "see" only one half of an opaque 3D object (transparent objects are relatively rare in most natural environments). As a result, our retina does not provide direct information about whole 3D objects. It does, however, contain some depth information in addition to the 2D retinal positions of various features of the objects. This partial information about depth is represented by the ".5" in Marr's "2.5D" label. Marr explains the significance and nature of the 2.5D sketch in his table 1.1 (Marr, 1982, p. 37) where it can be seen that the 2.5D sketch precedes the stage at which a 3D shape is represented. This means that in Marr's theory, shape is perceived by "taking orientation (or slant) into account," the same kind of misguided explanation that has dominated thinking about the perception of shape for centuries. N.B. that by introducing his 2.5D representation, Marr was able to ignore the importance of figure–ground organization, which provides the contour used to establish the 2D shape of the object's representation in the retinal image. By doing this, Marr assumed that figure–ground organization was not necessary for providing the percept of the 3D shape of an object. In his words, "most early visual processes extract information about the visible surfaces *directly*, without particular regard to whether they happen to be part of a horse, or a man, or a tree" (Marr, 1982, p. 272). How could he get away with this so long after the Gestalt psychologists had revolutionized perception by demonstrating the importance of figure–ground organization? Julesz (1960) had prepared the way by using random-dot stereograms in which figure–ground organization cannot be performed because the random-dot images do not provide any information about the contours of any objects. In the absence of any contours, 3D surfaces were perceived by applying binocular disparity *directly* to individual points and features of the retinal images.

Once depth and orientation of each part of the surface are computed, a 3D shape is perceived and segregated from its background.

Here we see that Marr, like Gibson, simplified the perceptual processing involved in 3D shape perception. Neither Marr nor Gibson believed that they needed Gestalt rules of perceptual organization in their theories, and each assumed that the 3D representation characterized by surfaces of objects is produced very early in perceptual processing. The difference is that Marr knew that computations are required to arrive at 3D representations, but Gibson thought that they were not. In Marr's theory, 3D shape is derived from the orientation of edges and surfaces. As a result, shape is treated the same way as all other spatial properties of the environment. For example, the shape of a box is treated in Marr's theory the same way as a set of six rectangles or as a set of twelve edges in 3D. Consider figure 3.2. Figure 3.2a is a Necker cube, an image of a wire cube. Figure 3.2b is an image of a polygonal line connecting the vertices of a cube (figure 3.2a) in a haphazard order. These two figures look quite different, and a successful theory of shape is likely to treat these figures very differently. However, Marr's theory does not. Both (a) and (b) are treated the same way. Marr begins by using depth cues such as binocular disparity or motion parallax to compute the 3D orientations of the edges in both figures. The result of

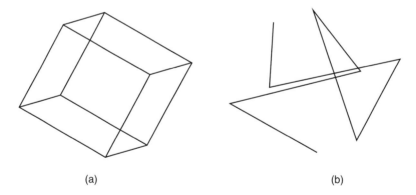

(a)   (b)

Figure 3.2
(a) A Necker cube. (b) An image of a polygonal line produced by connecting the vertices of the cube in a haphazard order. Note that (a) is more likely to be perceived as a 3D object than (b). Furthermore, "Necker-cube" depth reversal is easily observed in (a), but not in (b). Finally, the cube in (a) will show shape constancy, that is, it will be seen as a cube regardless of the direction from which it is viewed.

this computation is what he called a "2.5D" sketch. Once the 2.5D sketch is computed, the 3D shapes of these two objects are represented in the viewer-centered coordinate system. The next, and final, step in Marr's theory changes the frame of reference, from viewer-centered to object-centered. In Marr's theory, the representations of these two objects are equally good despite the fact that one is perceived as having shape and the other is not. Clearly, the Necker cube (a) is different in a number of ways from the unstructured wire object (b). Specifically, the differences are (i) shape constancy is achieved in (a), but not in (b), when binocular disparity or other depth cues are available (Rock & DiVita, 1987; Pizlo & Stevenson, 1999; Pizlo et al., 2005); (ii) a 3D object is perceived in (a), but not in (b), when depth cues are *not* available; and (iii) a reversal of depth is easily observed in (a), but not in (b). These differences are related to the fundamental fact that the image in (a) has shape properties emerging from the operation of figure–ground organization, but the image in (b) does not. Figure 3.3 shows that the same applies when the Necker cube is distorted. Figure 3.4 shows that it still applies even when the object is much more complex.[6]

In the next figure, figure 3.5, the difference between the two objects has been reduced considerably. How was this done? Symmetry was introduced. Symmetry made the polygonal line begin to look like the shape of a real

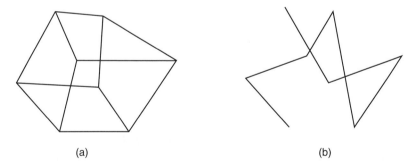

(a)   (b)

Figure 3.3
(a) An image of a nonrectangular box. (b) An image of a polygonal line produced by connecting the vertices of the box in a haphazard order. Note that (a) is more likely to be perceived as a 3D object than (b). Furthermore, "Necker-cube type" of depth reversal is easily observed in (a), but not in (b). Finally, the box in (a) will show shape constancy, that is, it will be seen as (approximately) the same box regardless of the direction from which it is viewed.

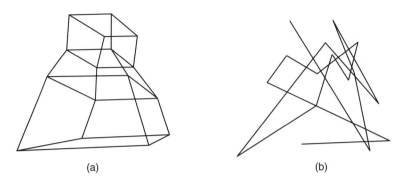

(a)   (b)

Figure 3.4
A complex object (a) and a wire object (b). The wire connects the vertices of the object in (b) in a random order.

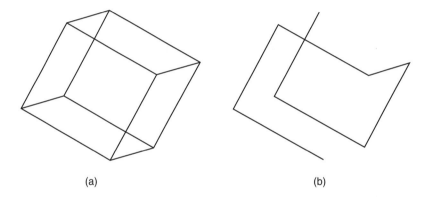

(a)   (b)

Figure 3.5
(a) A Necker cube. (b) An image of a polygonal line produced by connecting the vertices of the cube in an order that makes it easier to form groups of vertices that correspond to individual faces and that encompass a volume. Now, both (a) and (b) are perceived as 3D objects, and both lead to "Necker-cube" depth reversal.

object. It begins to resemble a Marcel Breuer dining chair. This polygonal line can be made even more like this chair by changing the order in which the points are connected. This is shown in figure 3.6. The polygonal line in figure 3.6b looks quite a bit like a 3D object. It is even capable of depth reversal. So, what emerges when we consider these figures (figures 3.2–3.6)? This series proceeded by introducing the properties that facilitate the operation of figure–ground organization, the Gestalt grouping principle, which is responsible for creating shapes that represent objects separated

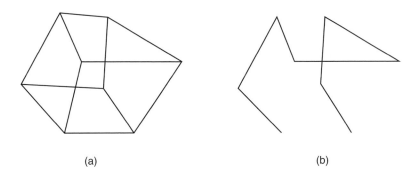

(a)   (b)

Figure 3.6
(a) An image of a nonrectangular box. (b) An image of a polygonal line produced by connecting the vertices of the box in an order that makes it easier to form groups of vertices that correspond to individual faces and that encompass a volume. Both (a) and (b) are perceived as 3D objects, and both lead to "Necker-cube" depth reversal.

from their background. It is this perceptual organizing principle that is critical for making it possible for a simple line drawing to look like a 3D shape that has volume and surfaces. The 3D geometrical features of the object, such as the orientations of its surfaces, which are represented in Marr's 2.5D sketch, are less important than the figure–ground organizing principles that operate in the 2D representation of a scene (its retinal image). Marr ignored figure-ground organization for two reasons. First, no one knew how to model it. Second, Julesz had demonstrated with his random-dot stereograms that a 3D percept can be produced by contourless images. However, figures 3.2–3.6 clearly show that Marr's approach, which produces 3D shape from a 2.5D sketch, contains a fatal flaw. Namely, Marr's approach will not be able to model human vision in real scenes without incorporating the figure–ground organizing principle. Figure–ground organization cannot be ignored.

Once one recognizes the critical role of figure–ground organization, a 2D property, the only property available in the retinal representation of the 3D world, a question arises about the relation between the shape of a 2D representation and the shape of a 3D object. Namely, what kind of information is available for the visual nervous system to use to create a 3D percept? Only two kinds of information are available: specifically, a contour, and the region enclosed by the contour. Both are used by the visual system to reconstruct the surface and volume of the 3D percept. Once these sources of information are identified, the next question becomes how much information is provided by the shape of a 3D object on the retina. Shape, unlike all other visual properties, such as brightness, speed, or size, is very special. Shape is complex, and this complexity is almost never eliminated by perspective projection. This means that the shape of a 2D retinal image, as represented by its contour, usually contains a lot of information, in most cases, enough to permit the visual system to reconstruct a veridical 3D shape percept.

3.1.4 Representation and Recognition of 3D Shapes Involves 3D Models

The final stage in Marr's theory is forming a 3D model of a 3D shape after the 2.5D sketch is derived from the retinal image by using depth cues. The main difference between Marr's 3D model and his 2.5D sketch is that the 3D model uses an object-centered representation, which *does not* depend on the observer's viewpoint, whereas the 2.5D sketch uses a viewer-centered representation, which *does*. Marr correctly pointed out that recognition of 3D shape from an arbitrary viewing direction (i.e., shape constancy) must involve an object-centered representation. Marr also spelled out three aspects that characterized his 3D model. The first is the coordinate system used to represent the 3D shape. If a given 3D shape is to be recognized as the same regardless of the viewing direction, the shape should be expressed in a coordinate system based on some distinctive features such as the elongation and symmetry of the object (Rock, 1973; Palmer, 1985, 1999). Marr's second aspect is a set of primitives. Here, Marr proposes surface-based features, which are directly derived from a 2.5D sketch, as well as volumetric features. Volumetric features may be very simple, such as small cubes, or as complex as parts of objects, such as an animal's limbs. Note that, according to Marr's theory, volumetric features come in very late in visual processing. They come after 3D surfaces are described in the object-centered coordinate system. One can say that in Marr's theory, the percept deals with surfaces, but it does not deal with volumes. Volumes, in Marr's theory, reside in the observer's memory, where models of 3D shapes are stored.

Marr's third aspect is the spatial organization of these primitives. Marr argues that the organization should be "modular," representing the hierarchical relation of the entire 3D object to its parts. For example, a human body consists of several parts such as limbs, a torso, and a head. Each limb has two main components, lower and upper, connected by a joint (e.g., an elbow). The lower part (a forearm) has, in turn two parts, and so on (see Marr's figure 5.3).

In the next chapter, the reader will see how Marr's ideas were developed by Biederman (1987) in his recognition-by-components theory. Despite several common features, there are several important differences between Marr's and Biederman's approaches. Marr derived the 3D model of shape from a 2.5D sketch without figure–ground organization, whereas Biederman derived the 3D shape from features characterizing the retinal 2D shape *after* figure–ground organization has been accomplished. Marr's theory relies heavily on depth cues and makes minimal use of a simplicity principle ("depth cues," as used in this treatment, refers to visual information that can be used to compute spatially local properties of surfaces, such as distances from the observer, relative distances along the depth direction, and 3D orientations). Biederman's theory relies heavily on a simplicity principle and makes no use of depth cues. Marr treated shape as a higher order variable derived from depth, whereas Biederman assigned a unique status to shape. Marr's 3D model clearly was a precursor of modern theories of shape, but other features of Marr's theory, notably his emphasis on the 2.5D sketch and his neglect of figure–ground organization, did not allow him, or his followers, to take the next step, namely, to reconstruct 3D shape from the 2D retinal representation of the 3D object.

3.1.5 Marr's Failure to Emphasize Psychophysical Experiments with Human Observers

Marr was a theoretical neuroscientist by training, and his interest in vision was motivated by the remarkable achievements of biological systems, such as the human visual system. Marr, despite his appreciation of these achievements, clearly had a bias when it came to evaluating the relative importance of psychophysical vis-à-vis simulation results. He was willing to refer to existing psychophysical data to illustrate some of his claims and to justify some of the assumptions upon which he built his theories, but he stopped there. He did not perform new psychophysical experiments with human observers, the kind of experiments that were actually *essential* for testing his theories directly. According to Whitman Richards, Marr's collaborator, Marr's initial intention was to conduct psychophysical experiments concurrently with developing computational models of vision: "We realized [in 1976] that the 'three levels' of understanding could also be recast as a scientific protocol for attacking a vision problem: Step 1: propose a computational theory; Step 2: write an algorithm embodying the theory; Step 3: check out its (biological) merit with psychophysics (or neurophysiology)" (Richards, 1990, p. 2). This protocol was applied in the late 1970s to stereopsis. However, "unfortunately, over the course of the years, as the problems became harder, the enforcement of the 1–2–3 method became lax, and often we did not get closure when studying a problem" (Richards, 1990, p. 3). It is possible, perhaps even likely, that Marr would have performed all of the necessary psychophysical experiments had he lived longer. His untimely death at the young age of thirty-five interrupted his highly creative work. He had only worked on vision for about ten years, not nearly enough time to "enforce the 1–2–3 method" in more than a handful of cases. Marr began by concentrating on developing computational models, the area in which his main talents lay. He might have accomplished much less than he did if he had tried to do psychophysical experiments with human observers at the same time.

The results of a number of psychophysical experiments on shape perception were available when Marr began his work in the 1970s, but computational models of shape perception were not, so it is not surprising that Marr, who emphasized the need for using computational models in vision, began by trying to remedy this imbalance by concentrating on developing computational models without engaging in concurrent psychophysical experimentation. Marr's failure to do concurrent psychophysical experiments proved to be a serious flaw. It doomed his approach because Marr's paradigm was built on a very strong, but unwarranted, assumption about the relation between 3D surfaces and 3D shapes. Namely, he assumed that perceiving 3D *surfaces* was *necessary* for the perception of 3D *shape*. No matter how obvious this assumption appeared to be to Marr and his associates, it should have been tested in psychophysical experiments before being used to build computational models of shape perception. This should have been clear at the time because psychophysical results published by the neo-Gestaltists during the 1960s and 1970s had already suggested that this assumption was unwarranted (see chapter 2).

Why was a psychophysical experiment to test the primacy assumption about 3D surfaces critical when Marr began to formulate his theory of shape? It was critical because once it is assumed that the percept of surfaces is *necessary* for the percept of shape, it becomes obvious that shape *must* be based on the perception of depth because the perception of 3D surfaces is derived from depth cues. Recall that "depth cues" refers to the visual information that can be used to compute the spatially local properties of surfaces, namely, the distances from the observer, relative distances along the depth direction, and 3D orientations. However, as the reader already knows from the discussion in section 3.1.3, 3D surfaces can be perceived in the absence of depth cues. By way of a reminder, it is obvious that the surfaces and edges of a Necker cube are perceived as 3D only because they are surfaces and edges of a 3D shape percept, a percept that is derived from the operation of a simplicity principle. It is not derived from depth cues. One way to contrast this Necker cube example with Marr's theory is to realize that in this example, 3D surfaces are produced from the volume of an object, not the other way around. It follows that *3D surfaces can have a dual role in vision*: They can be derived from spatially local depth cues (as they are with unstructured, irregular objects, such as ragged rocks, potatoes, tree branches, and wire objects) or from the perceived 3D shape (as they are with structured objects, such as a Necker cube, human-made objects, and animals). To put it differently, a 3D shape can serve as a cue to 3D surface, but not the other way around. Marr overlooked this fact. Once the dual role of surfaces is recognized as a theoretical possibility, it immediately becomes clear that the shape perceived may not be predictable from the perceived surfaces. If the perceived shape cannot be predicted from the perceived surfaces, Marr's theory *must* be rejected. This is not difficult to test, so it is remarkable that this experiment was not performed during the 30 years that followed the introduction of Marr's computational theory of shape perception. Suitable experiments were performed only very recently by the present author and his colleagues (Li & Pizlo, 2006; Pizlo et al., 2006). They clearly showed that the perceived 3D shape cannot be predicted from the perceived 3D surfaces of the shape (see chapter 4 for details). Marr would have known that a completely different theory was needed if this psychophysical experiment had been performed 30 years earlier. Had this been done, the vision community might have concentrated on exploring the uniqueness of shape, rather than on trying to find weaknesses in the approach of those few, such as Biederman, who studied shape outside of the context of depth and surface perception.

3.1.6 The Relative Importance of Shape Regularities and Cues to Depth

Consider objects that have some regularities, such as symmetries. From the computational point of view, a vision system may proceed in two ways. The first is to reconstruct the 3D shape by using the symmetries that are present in the object. This is the approach taken by this author. The second is to reconstruct the 3D shape from depth cues. This was Marr's approach. Note that this approach ends up reconstructing symmetries of the object from depth cues. This is clearly a roundabout method. *Why ignore symmetry, and other regularities, when they are "there"? Depth cues are never perfectly reliable, so the reconstruction with depth cues will be less accurate than reconstruction without them.* It follows that the human visual system would do well by using the first approach. It does. The remaining question is how many objects "out there" have regularities. This is an open question that should be answered by a "statistical survey of ecological stimulus representativeness," as advocated by Brunswik (1956, chapters 8–10). It seems to me that most, if not all, objects that have functional significance to us actually have regularities, such as symmetries. If this is the case, then the theory of shape perception proposed in this book applies to human shape perception in our everyday life.

Now that we understand the uniqueness of shape and the importance of figure–ground organization in producing a 3D percept of shape, it is obvious that Marr's 2.5D sketch is not the best level at which to start to model human shape perception. Unfortunately, the pervasive influence of Marr's approach postponed serious consideration of figure–ground organization until recently. Why was Marr's approach so influential? Marr's approach was introduced shortly after Julesz (1960) made a big impression on the vision science community with his random-dot stereograms. Julesz' stereograms made it possible to see 3D surfaces and 3D shapes without contours in the retinal image. This fact, of course, does not rule out the importance of contours in shape perception. After all, once the stereograms are fused and the 3D surfaces perceived, the image contours can be inferred and used to produce the 3D shape percept. In other words, there is no reason why binocular disparity might not serve as a cue to contours, the same way shading, texture, and motion do (Regan, 2000; Knill, 2001). Is this the mechanism the visual system normally uses, or is it an exception to its normal mode of action? It is difficult to answer this question directly at our stage of knowledge, but it seems likely to be an exception if only because random-dot stereograms could have exerted very little evolutionary pressure in our environment. Shapes derived from Julesz' stereograms were probably not perceived by anyone before 1960.

3.2   Reconstruction of 3D Shape from Shading, Texture, Binocular Disparity, Motion, and Multiple Views

At about the same time Marr's (1982) book appeared, a set of computational vision papers was published as volume 17 of *Artificial Intelligence* (1981; this volume is also available as a book edited by Brady, 1981). These papers illustrate how the geometry of surfaces described in the 2.5D sketch can be reconstructed from different types of visual cues. This work used a variety of visual cues, including shading, motion, texture, and binocular disparity, together with assumptions about the surfaces and objects to be reconstructed. The most prominent assumptions (constraints) were smoothness of the reconstructed surface and rigidity of the reconstructed point set. Working within Marr's paradigm, these studies did not include figure–ground organization. Without figure–ground organization, retinal shape is not available, which means that shape invariants and shape constraints have no place. In this case, the *only* way to produce 3D shapes is to reconstruct the visible surfaces as Marr proposed and then "take their orientation into account" to produce 3D shapes. If shape invariants and shape constraints were allowed to operate, the 3D shape itself could be recognized or reconstructed. Both could be accomplished without "taking the orientation of the surfaces into account." Thus, allowing figure–ground organization increases the number of options; takes advantage of the special virtue inherent in shape, namely, complexity; and provides a model that can actually create a 3D percept from a 2D image. Figure–ground organization was not incorporated in this large body of work, so only three papers from this set, those most relevant to shape, will be described here because it was clear that a significant advance in our understanding of shape perception could not emerge from this approach. The three were included primarily to give the reader a feel for what was going on at this stage of development of our current knowledge about shape, not because they were important to its development.

The first paper in this set analyzed the use of texture (Witkin, 1981). Witkin gave credit to Gibson (1950) for pointing out the importance of texture and texture gradients, but he also indicated that Gibson underestimated the difficulty in using texture in the case of real images. Gibson hoped that there is a simple quantity that can be used to characterize a texture gradient, a quantity that could give a direct measure of the surface slant and tilt at each point of the surface. In the case of realistic images, there is no such quantity because texture is never perfectly regular. Once there is variability in the geometrical properties of texture, one *must* use statistical methods, such as maximum likelihood, to estimate the surface geometry on the basis of data sampled from many parts of the surface.

The second paper in this series analyzed surface contours (Stevens, 1981). Using results from differential geometry, Stevens analyzed properties of geodesics and of lines of curvature (see Hilbert & Cohn-Vossen, 1952, and Koenderink, 1995, for excellent reviews of the differential geometry of surfaces). Stevens pointed out that for cylindrical surfaces, the lines of curvatures are both planar curves and geodesics. If we can assume that image contours are planar geodesics, we can (under some additional assumptions) reconstruct the geometry of the surface (Stevens, 1981, 1986). Despite the fact that surfaces of natural objects are never exactly cylindrical, they are close enough to cylindrical to make Stevens' method useful.

Finally, the paper by Barrow and Tenenbaum (1981) analyzed the role of both visual cues and a simplicity principle in explaining the percept of visible surfaces. These authors used smoothness, planarity, and the minimum variance of angles constraints to reconstruct shapes of polyhedral objects. It is worth pointing out that their explanation of the percept of polyhedra did not fit within Marr's paradigm because the minimum variance of angles constraint can only be applied to an organized figure (the retinal shape of a figure). Barrow and Tennebaum's approach was subsequently used by Marill (1991) and Leclerc and Fischler (1992) in their computer graphics algorithms, as well as by the present author (Pizlo, 2001) in his model of shape perception formulated within the framework of inverse problems.

A number of other studies on shape and space perception appeared in this period. They used constraints, but not those requiring figure–ground organization. These studies include reconstruction of 2D and 3D motion with the application of smoothness constraints (e.g., Hildreth, 1984); reconstruction of surfaces from shading (Horn, 1975, 1977; Ikeuchi & Horn, 1981), again with the use of a smoothness constraint applied to surfaces; and computation of structure (shape) from motion with the use of a rigidity constraint (Ullman, 1979; Longuet-Higgins, 1981). These two studies on what is called "structure from motion" have been especially influential in the study of shape perception.

The first, and more influential of the two, was Ullman's (1979), who developed a computational model to explain the KDE described by Wallach and O'Connell (1953). Recall that Wallach and O'Connell demonstrated that viewing the shadow of a 3D rotating rigid object can give rise to the percept of a 3D rotating rigid object. Furthermore, they described conditions in which the percept of a 3D rigid object could not be obtained. They stopped short of providing a theory of the KDE. Ullman picked up this problem and developed an algorithm for reconstructing a 3D object from a sequence of 2D images. He assumed an orthographic projection from the 3D scene to the 2D image (an orthographic projection is an approximation to perspective projection; it assumes that the projecting lines are orthogonal to the image plane). Ullman further assumed that the correspondences of points across images were known. Based on these assumptions, Ullman showed that given three views of four non-coplanar points rotating in a rigid fashion in 3D space, it is possible to compute the depth of each point (its relative distance to the image). This is Ullman's well-known "structure from motion theorem." Note that Ullman's algorithm, by assigning depths to retinal points, provides a 2.5D sketch. The shape of the retinal image is not required, so figure–ground organization is irrelevant. Ullman's 3D "shape," represented by the points in 3D, is established after their depths are computed. Ullman's approach raises a couple of questions. Mathematically, his algorithm works, but this by itself does not mean (i) that it can be used to reconstruct the shapes of *real* objects in *real* environments or (ii) that it describes how the human visual system produces the 3D percept of shape. The first question arises because of the fact that there is always noise in real images of the 3D environment. Ullman's reconstruction method does not work reliably in the presence of noise because the reconstruction result is computationally unstable. This, by itself, implies that it cannot be used as a model of how humans acquire shape information from motion. There are also other problems. First, the human observer's ability to see 3D shape based on motion depends critically on the nature of the objects. Specifically, when human observers are asked to discriminate shapes of 3D objects based on motion, they can do it very well, but only when structured objects are used, not when 3D polygonal lines are used (Pizlo & Stevenson, 1999). There is nothing in Ullman's algorithm that can account for this difference. Furthermore, rigid objects that can be reconstructed by Ullman's algorithm may or may not be perceived as rigid by human observers (Pizlo & Salach-Golyska, 1995). Conversely, objects that are nonrigid, and are interpreted as such by Ullman's algorithm, may actually be perceived as rigid by human observers (Pizlo, Li, & Francis, 2005). These differences between Ullman's algorithm and the percepts of human observers can be eliminated if figure–ground organization is used before the 3D shape is reconstructed.

The second influential study on structure from motion was done by Longuet-Higgins (1981). He formulated a mathematical method for reconstructing 3D spatial positions of points from perspective images taken by two calibrated cameras (see appendix C, section C.2, for a definition of perspective projection).[7] When two cameras view a 3D scene simultaneously, the conditions emulate those of a "binocular observer." If only one camera is used, and it takes two images, each from a different viewing direction, the conditions emulate those used to study the KDE. Mathematically, these two cases are equivalent. However, perceptually, they may not be equivalent because the position and orientation of one eye relative to another is not arbitrary in a binocular observer. Furthermore, analyzing two images obtained sequentially requires the use of memory, whereas analyzing two images obtained simultaneously does not. Longuet-Higgins did not make any assumptions about the relative positions of the two cameras, so his algorithm can be treated as a structure-from-motion algorithm, although Longuet-Higgins speculated that his algorithm could be used as a model of binocular vision, as well. Longuet-Higgins' method is analogous to that of Ullman in that it reconstructs depths of points from motion information. Figure–ground organization is not used. Longuet-Higgins showed that images of eight points can be used to compute eight parameters in an "essential matrix" representing the relation between image points in two perspective views.[8] Note that only six of those eight parameters are independent. These independent parameters correspond to the six degrees of freedom of a rigid body in 3D. After the fundamental matrix is computed, the 3D rotation and translation between the two cameras is reconstructed. This allows the computation of 3D Euclidean coordinates of the points. Longuet-Higgins' algorithm is similar to Ullman's. They both provide a mathematical solution to the structure-from-motion problem. The algorithms are, however, quite different. Ullman's algorithm requires three images and uses an orthographic approximation to perspective projection. Longuet-Higgins' algorithm requires only two images, and it uses perspective projection. Despite these differences, these two algorithms suffer from exactly the same problems: inability to deal effectively with visual noise and to predict the percepts of human observers. It seems likely that these algorithms have the same problems because of the same reason. Namely, they do not make use of figure–ground organization.

To summarize, computational methods formulated within Marr's paradigm did not lead to models of human shape perception. They also did not solve this problem for machine vision because of their inability to deal with real images. Clearly, Marr's decision to substitute the 2.5D sketch for figure–ground organization was a dead end. Once the limitations of Marr's approach became clear, two new classes of methods were introduced in the middle and late 1980s. The first group was based on invariants of projective transformation. The second group was based on the formalism called "inverse problems." Both were quite promising, although neither led to the solution of Marr's "big problem" of formulating a computational theory of a general-purpose vision system.

3.3 Recognition of Shape Based on Invariants

Many think that Gibson introduced the idea that shape and space perception involves "invariants" because he spoke about "invariants" throughout his career (Gibson, 1950, 1966, 1979). However, few realize that for Gibson, "invariants" was only a slogan. He provided no mathematical treatment of what he meant by "invariants," and he frequently misused the colloquial term (see appendix C, section C.5, for a review of groups of transformations and their invariants). Furthermore, Gibson's claims about which properties of the 3D environment are, or are not, "invariant" when they are represented on the retina have been shown to be incorrect (e.g., see

Witkin's, 1981, discussion of texture gradients; Hay's, 1966, discussion of shape from motion of 2D figures; and Ullman's, 1980, discussion of shape from motion of 3D objects). Gibson probably derived his lifelong commitment to "invariants" from his recognition of the fact that shape constancy is of fundamental importance. It allows human beings to perceive 3D objects veridically. Gibson felt that it was particularly important to emphasize veridicality because many of his contemporaries devoted all of their efforts to studying illusions, failures of veridicality. Gibson's contribution to shape perception, however, did not go beyond this. He did not provide a theory of either shape or space perception. Note that he was not in a position to do this even if he had wanted to because he believed that the veridical reconstruction of Euclidean properties can be done by using projective invariants. Mathematically, this makes no sense, whatsoever. Projective invariants *cannot* be used to reconstruct Euclidean properties (see appendix C, section C.6, for a review of projective invariants and their use in machine vision applications).

What, if anything, did Gibson's emphasis on "invariants" contribute to perception? His emphasis did contribute, but the contribution was much less general than he and his students realized. Consider first where he did make an important contribution. Gibson's idea of "direct perception," based on invariants, works in auditory perception. A melody (a distal stimulus) can be specified by ratios of frequencies of tones (the tune) and by ratios of time intervals (the rhythm). Gibson correctly pointed out that both ratios are preserved in the proximal stimulus (Gibson, 1966, chapter 5). This means that a melody is constant at three levels: in the distal stimulus, in the proximal stimulus, and in the percept. In other words, a melody is invariant in its transformation from distal to proximal stimulus, allowing the auditory system to perceive the melody "directly" (to "pick it up"— Gibson, 1966, p. 89). Only a few simple computations are required. Thus, "direct" perception is possible in audition, but not in vision, particularly not in the perception of 3D shapes. With 3D shapes, no ratios are preserved in the proximal stimulus. The 3D distal stimulus is projected to a 2D retinal image. In order to perceive shapes veridically (to achieve shape constancy), the visual system must *reconstruct* the 3D shape. It cannot simply "pick it up."

Now that we know that invariants do not apply to vision in the way Gibson claimed, we turn to an additional problem in his approach. Gibson also confused the colloquial and mathematical meanings of the term "invariant." It is easy to confuse the two because *mathematical invariants*, superficially, look as though they could provide a natural basis for explaining *shape constancy*. Note that shape constancy is a "perceptual invariant" in the sense that *the perceived shape remains constant ("invariant"), despite changes in the retinal shape*. However, a problem arises when you consider what a mathematician means when he or she says "invariant." In mathematics, a given feature is invariant when it is *not changed* by a given transformation. For example, shape is invariant under rigid motions (translations and rotations), but it is *not invariant* when projected on the retina.[9] The projection of an object to its retinal image *changes* its shape, but in perception, the perceived shape of an object is said to be "invariant" *despite* changes of its shape on the retina. Thus, the statement that "shape is a perceptual invariant" leads to confusion, unless the definition of "shape" or the definition of "invariant" (or both) are changed. Clearly, we must begin with unambiguous definitions of the terms "invariant" and "shape" before we can discuss how "invariants" can be used in models of shape perception. However, even before we define "invariants" and "shape," we have to clarify what we mean by "models" and "theories" that have been, and/or could be, used to "explain" the perception of shape.

3.3.1 Models, Theories, and Plausible Explanations

The meanings of the terms "theory," "model," and "explanation" changed throughout the period when progress was being made in the study of shape perception. The ways in which these terms were used in the past, and how they are used now, have to be appreciated before one can understand why some of what were called "theories" and "explanations" dozens of years ago do not meet contemporary standards. Not everyone appreciates the importance of these changes of meanings even today. Failure to do so can lead to disagreements and confusion about what constitutes progress in the study of shape and what does not (what will be called "milestones" and "millstones" at the end of this book). The meanings of such important terms as "theory," "model," and "explanation" have varied a lot during the last 100 years. The standards for what it means to formulate a theory, to model, or to explain something improved during the twentieth century, particularly since the end of World War II. The standards have improved in the sense that these terms are now based on relatively precise, unambiguous formalisms. These improvements have made it clear why earlier uses of these terms proved to be, by contemporary standards, unfruitful. For example, one of the main reasons why Gibson's approach did not lead to a plausible theory of shape perception is that Gibson's "theorizing" never went beyond the stage of potentially interesting ideas. Gibson, writing in the second half of the twentieth century understood terms such as "theory" and "explanation" the same way psychologists had understood them for at least a half century before he published. Today, what Gibson and his contemporaries called a "theory" would be called a "hypothesis," at best. What do we expect the terms "theory" and "explanation" to mean today?

A "theory" of a natural phenomenon, such as shape perception, should lead to an "explanation" of the phenomenon. There is no universally accepted definition of what is meant by an "explanation" that can be applied in all fields of science (Braithwaite, 1955; Nagel, 1961). However, in shape perception, it is quite widely accepted that a plausible "explanation" should provide a description of how the information available on the retina is used by the human being's visual system to produce a veridical percept of shape. In other words, what I will call a "plausible" explanation is one that describes the computational mechanisms involved in producing a veridical percept of shape. This plausible explanation will take the form of a "computational model." It will be "plausible" because it produces the same result as the visual system, namely, it reconstructs the 3D shape from its 2D retinal representation. It "perceives shape" as it is perceived by a human observer, and it does this with a wide variety of realistic images, images that contain occlusions and visual noise that are prominent features of natural scenes. I am describing my approach to "explanation" because alternative approaches such as describing a relationship or correlation between some stimulus and the response to it, the kind of "black-box explanations" favored by behaviorists and connectionists in the past, will not do today. For example, it is not sufficient to "explain" shape perception by claiming that the observer has learned to associate shading, texture, and/or motion with memory traces of a retinal image and consequent actions, as Hebb (1949) in the middle of the twentieth century. and other later-day empiricists have done (see section 2.5). A satisfying, plausible, contemporary "explanation" would be based on a computational model of the processes underlying the perception of shape, rather than on verbal models like Gibson's or connectionist models based on what is now called a "Hebbian rule." Hebb's (1949) "model," of course, like most others of the period, was only verbal. It hypothesized that repetitions of fixation positions during scanning eye movements among various features in the visual array (mainly corners) lead to establishment of what was called a "phase sequence." This was Hebb's name for the neural engram that "represented" a particular "shape" in the brain. These engrams, the memories of sensorimotor learning, allowed a human observer to recognize a particular feature pattern as a particular shape when it was present in the visual array. The connectionist modelers, when they developed mathematical models to handle perceptual as well as other kinds of learning, chose to honor Hebb, rather than James (1890) or Dewey (1896) by referring to "Hebb's rule." "Hebb's rule" could just as aptly be called "Dewey's rule."

Developing a computational model that can simulate the mechanisms responsible for some perceptual property has been accepted as the "gold standard" since the 1970s when Marr and his group introduced this approach in the field of vision. Marr made it clear that a computational model is critical. Without it, a theory may have a number of hidden assumptions, assumptions that the theory's author may not appreciate. *Only after a theory (verbal or mathematical) is reformulated as a computational model, which can be tested in simulations using realistic stimuli, will it be possible to decide whether the particular computational theory can explain shape constancy.* In other words, a computational theory can describe what has been computed, and these computations, which are based on the 2D retinal image in the observer's eye, should lead to the veridical perception of the shape of the 3D object that produced this 2D image on the observer's retina. *If a computational model of shape perception does not lead to shape constancy, it cannot be a plausible description of the perceptual mechanisms underlying shape perception because human observers are known to achieve shape constancy under naturalistic as well as under many impoverished stimulating conditions.*

The arguments presented above are based on the observation that there is an intrinsic relationship between the property called "shape" and shape constancy. Namely, shape constancy is the sine qua non of shape. To put it in everyday parlance, shape is not perceived if shape constancy fails. Note that this almost never happens in everyday life. It follows that *it is not meaningful to talk about shape and shape perception without including, even emphasizing, shape constancy.* This point is essential. It is commonly agreed that "shape" refers to those geometrical properties of objects that are independent of the object's orientation relative to the observer (Marr, 1982). It follows that the only way one can be sure that one is studying shape perception, as opposed to the perception of depth, shading, motion, natural scenes, and so forth, is to study shape constancy—that is, to study the observer's ability to perceive shapes veridically despite changes in the viewing orientation of the object relative to the observer. Testing the effect of viewing distance, illumination conditions, surface texture, binocular disparity, and so forth, on the perception of objects does not, in itself, address the perception of shape or shape constancy. The manipulation of such variables falls into the literature supporting "taking into account" explanations of shape perception, a literature that has led nowhere to date. *There are no stimulus properties that can be attributed to shape beyond those that can be demonstrated in shape constancy experiments.* This statement is of fundamental importance. It was used by this author to choose the material that would be included in this book. Only those experiments and theories that contribute to our understanding of shape constancy have been discussed in detail. Others have only been mentioned or left out entirely.

Achieving shape constancy is computationally very difficult. At present, there is no machine vision system that can solve this task as well as a human observer does. Note, however, that there have been a number of theories and models in the human literature claiming to have explained shape constancy. Had these models been plausible, they could have been used to produce a machine vision system that worked as well as the human visual system, a system that achieves shape constancy easily. Existing machine vision systems are not plausible because they cannot achieve shape constancy. It follows that computational modeling gives the scientist interested in shape perception a distinct advantage because using computational models, tested with realistic simulations, eliminates the difficulties inherent in choosing a plausible theory by using Popper's (1979) falsification criterion or by using something akin to Occam's razor for "model selection" (Pitt, Myung, & Zhang, 2002), the only techniques available before computational modeling was introduced into visual science.

We turn next to explaining which invariants can, and which invariants cannot, be used in models of shape perception now that we (i) know how the term "invariants" came to be employed; (ii) have considered the history of changing meanings of such basic terms as "theory," model," and "explanation" during the last century; and (iii) have explained the author's reasons for preferring computational models over other approaches to the study of shape perception.

3.3.2 Projective Invariants Cannot Explain Shape Constancy

First, consider how a mathematician applies invariants to shape constancy. As pointed out just above, shape is not invariant in the projection to the retinal image. Specifically, ratios of distances, as well as angles, change. What does not change, however, is a cross ratio of areas. This cross ratio is called a "projective invariant." Thus, the statement "Shape is a perceptual invariant" is understood by a mathematician as implying that shape is characterized by projective invariants. You will see that this approach, despite its precision and elegance, *cannot* lead to a satisfactory explanation of shape constancy. In fact, you will see that if the visual system itself had adopted such an approach, our ability to perceive the visual world veridically would be quite limited, much more than it actually is. There is an additional problem. Namely, projective invariants can only be applied to 2D shapes. They cannot be used to explain 3D shape constancy.[10] The significance of this limitation, which has only been appreciated recently, will be discussed, in detail, after limitations inherent in using projective invariants are explained.

Projective invariants have received considerable attention in machine vision since 1988, when Weiss published a paper applying projective invariants to shape recognition. The application of projective invariants to four simple shapes is illustrated in figure 3.7. A pentagon, (a), and its two

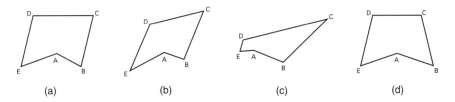

Figure 3.7
Pentagons (a), (b), and (c) are projectively equivalent and are characterized by the following cross ratios: (0.80, 0.32). The pentagon in (d) is projectively different from the other two. Its cross ratios are (1.75, 0.68).

projective images, (b) and (c), are shown (recall that a projective transformation is a product of two or more perspective transformations (see appendix C, section C.7, for a discussion of differences between perspective and projective transformations). The projective invariant used consists of two cross ratios of corresponding areas of triangles (see appendix A, section A.3, for definitions of these invariants). The values of the two cross ratios are identical for the three pentagons, which means that each is a projective transformation of any of the other two.

These three figures are projectively the same, but they do not "look" the same. The reader surely agrees. The shapes in figure 3.7a and 3.7b look similar—(b) looks like a slanted (a)—but the shapes in (a) and (c) look different. Remember that, *projectively*, all three are the same. Furthermore, the shape in figure 3.7d is projectively different from (a), but it looks similar to it. Clearly, projective invariants cannot explain either shape similarity or shape constancy.[11] An even clearer illustration of the limitations of projective invariants is provided by quadrilaterals. Specifically, according to projective invariants, there is *only one* convex quadrilateral (Pizlo, Rosenfeld, & Weiss, 1997a)! In other words, all convex quadrilaterals, like those in figure 3.8, are projectively the same. They should be perceived as having the same shape. Are they?

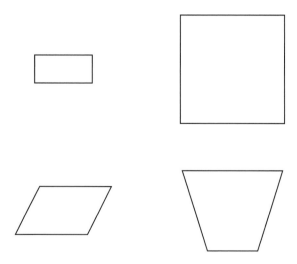

Figure 3.8
Several convex quadrilaterals. They are projectively but not perceptually equivalent.

This limitation of projective invariants has often been overlooked or considered unimportant. How could something so striking have been considered to be unimportant? Consider several shapes that are actually projectively different, like the three polygons in figure 3.9. Polygons like these never produce identical retinal images. Recall that projective invariants are also invariants of a perspective projection to the retina because a perspective projection is a special case of a projective transformation (see appendix C, section C.7). It follows that applying projective invariants to retinal images, rather than to shapes themselves, as was done in figure 3.7, could make it possible for the visual system to discriminate these three pentagons. This possibility is why one could overlook the limitations of projective invariants. However, note that the human visual system does not work this way. It can discriminate not only shapes that are projectively different, like those in figure 3.9, but also some shapes that are projectively identical, like those in figure 3.8. Put simply, if projective invariants were used by the visual system, we would not be able to distinguish a pizza box from a shoe box, so, despite the elegance and precision inherent in using projective invariants, this approach is not nearly as good as the visual system we have. Other kinds of invariants are required. What might they be? The next two sections describe examples of new invariants that seem to be moving us in the right direction.[12]

3.3.3   An Explanation of Shape Constancy Requires New Invariants

These new invariants derive from an appreciation of the fact that *perspective* projection plays an important role in shape constancy. They were

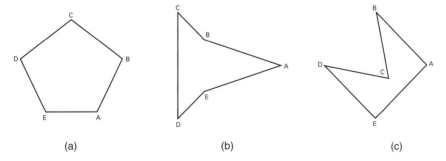

(a)   (b)   (c)

Figure 3.9
Three polygons that are projectively different. Projective invariants can be used to recognize these polygons from their perspective images. Their values are (a) 2.83, 1.65; (b) 0.83, 1.04; (c) 0.33, –1.00.

formulated to explain Stavrianos' (1945) results on shape constancy with 2D shapes oriented arbitrarily in 3D space (see chapter 1). Prior to the formulation of *perspective* invariants, Stavrianos' results were mysterious. They only made sense when the role of perspective projection in shape constancy was appreciated. The problem the visual system needs to solve when this question is asked is illustrated in figure 3.10. When viewed from a normal reading distance, with the line of sight orthogonal to (at a right angle with respect to) the plane of the figure, the retinal image of (b) is a perspective image of a slanted (a). The viewing distance and viewing direc-

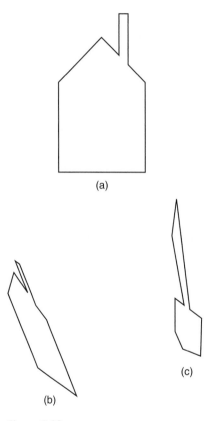

Figure 3.10
When the observer views the polygon (b) from a distance five times larger than the size of (b), with the line of sight orthogonal to the figure and with the fixation point at the center, the retinal image of (b) is a valid image of a slanted polygon (a), and it looks like a slanted (a). The polygon (c) is a projective image of (a), and it does not look like a slanted (a) (from Pizlo & Salach-Golyska, 1995).

tion are important now. They were not important earlier, because this is the first time we are talking about *perspective projection* and its consequences on the retina (see appendix C, section C.8, for a detailed discussion of a geometrical model of image formation). If the viewing distance was much shorter than normal, or if the line of sight was not orthogonal to the plane of the figure, the retinal image of (b) would not be a perspective image of a slanted (a). Instead, it would be a projective image of (a). Under such viewing conditions, (b) may not look like a slanted (a). However, when the reader looks at (b) from a normal viewing distance, with the line of sight orthogonal to the plane of the figure, (b) *does look like* a slanted (a), which means that shape constancy has been achieved. Invariants are needed to account for these two different percepts. Once such invariants are in place, they will be able to account for the fact that the retinal image of (c), when (c) is viewed from a normal reading distance, is *not* a perspective image of a slanted (a), and it is not perceived as such. In fact, (c) is a projective image of a slanted (a). One does not expect shape constancy under such conditions so it is not surprising that it is not observed. Clearly, with perspective images, shape constancy can be achieved, implying that *persp*ective invariants are involved. Recall that *proj*ective invariants cannot be effective here. When projective invariants are used, all three figures, (a), (b), and (c), are the same despite the way they look to us. These new invariants, called "perspective invariants," were introduced by Pizlo and Rosenfeld (1992) and tested in psychophysical experiments by Pizlo (1994) and Pizlo and Salach-Golyska (1995).[13] Invariants of a 2D perspectivity are explained in appendix C, section C.9.1.

The next section discusses shape constancy for solid objects. In this section another new type of invariant, as well as a new definition of shape, will be introduced.

3.3.4 Shape Constancy for Solid Objects—New Invariants and a New Definition of Shape

The first clear statement that projective invariants cannot be applied to recognition of a 3D shape from a single 2D image was presented by Burns et al. (1990). This limitation is directly related to the fact that a transformation from a 3D scene to a 2D retina is a many-to-one transformation. We now know, however, from the work of Sugihara (1986) and others (described in the beginning of this chapter) that a single 2D image makes it possible

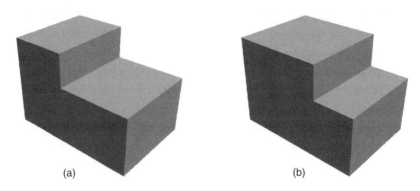

(a)   (b)

Figure 3.11
The objects in (a) and (b) are projectively different, and they can be discriminated by Rothwell's (1995) model-based invariants (produced using 3DS Max/Autodesk).

to discriminate among many 3D objects, as long as one is able to restrict the class of objects of interest. Consider the two polyhedral objects in figure 3.11. The reader surely agrees that (a) and (b) look different. And indeed, (a) and (b) are images of two different 3D objects. Sugihara's method for polyhedra can be used to verify this statement. The fact that a single 2D image allows one to discriminate two 3D objects, as shown in figure 3.11, implies that 2D images contain some useful "invariant" properties. Observations like this led Rothwell et al. (1993) to formulate a new class of invariants called "model-based invariants" for polyhedral objects. Rothwell (1995) extended this work by formulating projective model-based invariants for rotationally symmetrical objects with smooth surfaces ("solids of revolution"). Details of these methods are presented in appendix C, section C.10. Here, only a brief treatment of model-based invariants for polyhedra will be provided.

Rothwell considered polyhedra where all vertices were trihedral, like those in figure 3.11. That is, each vertex was an intersection of three planar faces. By using homogeneous coordinates (the method first used by Roberts, 1965), Rothwell was able to describe the (i) relations among the faces of a given polyhedron, (ii) perspective projection of the polyhedron made with an uncalibrated camera, and (iii) contours in the image, using linear equations. He then eliminated the unknown parameters, obtaining new model-based projective invariants. They are called "model-based" because they can be applied only to a restricted family of 3D shapes, in this case, polyhedra. Much was made above of the fact that projective invariants are insensitive to projective transformations of an object. The same problem arises here with 3D projective invariants that we encountered with 2D projective invariants. 3D shapes that look different to us will be treated as the same when projective invariants are used.[14]

3.4   Poggio's Elaboration of Marr's Approach: The Role of Constraints in Visual Perception

It should be obvious to the reader by now that the main difficulty in achieving veridical perception of 3D shapes stems from the fact that the retinal image is 2D. The visual system has to find a way of either reconstructing the missing depth information or solving the 3D problem without making use of information about depth. The first approach was adopted by Marr (1982), who introduced and emphasized the importance of what he called a "2.5D representation" in which depth is represented, albeit not completely (see sections 3.1 and 3.2). In the second approach, depth was ignored by those who used "invariants" to recognize shapes. We have seen that recognition based on projective invariants fell far short of what the human visual system can actually do. Perspective invariants provide a much better explanation of human shape recognition, but they cannot explain the perception of unfamiliar 3D shapes. Poggio, Torre, and Koch (1985) built on Marr's approach, which was designed to deal not only with familiar but also with unfamiliar 3D shapes (i) by emphasizing the importance of the 2.5D representation, which contains information about depth, and (ii) by assigning importance to the role of a priori constraints in producing the 2.5D sketch.

Poggio et al. (1985) began by pointing out that some of the assumptions, such as the rigidity of an object or the smoothness of a surface, that Marr incorporated in his computational model are not merely tools or tricks invoked to make the reconstruction of depth easier. Instead, they are critical elements in a formalism called "regularization theory" (Tikhonov & Arsenin, 1977). Regularization theory provides the means for solving "inverse problems" in science and engineering. Problems like these begin with recognizing that they can be solved in two "directions": one called "forward" or "direct" and the other called "inverse." Solving a "forward" problem is accomplished by predicting data from a model. Solving an "inverse" problem is accomplished by developing a model on the basis of data. For a simple example of how this can be applied, consider a physical law, for example, Newton's second law of motion. The law says that when a force F acts on a mass m, it results in acceleration, a, of the object: $a = F/m$. Computation of a from this formula, based on values of F and m, represents solving a "forward" problem. Inferring the law itself from the values of a, m, and F represents solving an "inverse" problem. The distinction being made is analogous to the difference between deductive and inductive reasoning. Forward problems are usually easy to solve. Inverse problems are usually difficult. Specifically, they are "ill posed," that is, (i) no solution exists, (ii) more than one solution exists, or (iii) the solution may change arbitrarily in the presence of small changes of the data. Furthermore, the solution may be unstable in the presence of noise in the data. In this last case, a problem is called "ill conditioned." According to regularization theory, a unique and stable solution of an inverse problem can be produced by imposing "a priori constraints" on the family of possible solutions.

Note that in practice, scientists and engineers are rarely actually asked to solve "forward problems." Forward problems are always "solved" by the physical systems themselves, not by the scientists or engineers who collect the data about the systems' operation. These scientists and engineers are usually asked to solve "inverse" problems associated with the operation of these physical systems. In other words, they *infer* the models from the data they collected. Note, however, that there is always more than one model that can account for the collected data.[15] In other words, "inverse problems" are usually ill posed and ill conditioned.

Poggio et al. (1985) pointed out that this approach also applies to visual perception. A typical "forward" problem could be producing a 2D retinal image (data) of a 3D object (model). This is accomplished simply by using the established rules of geometrical optics. The "inverse" of this problem requires inferring a veridical percept of a 3D object from its 2D retinal image. This, like all inverse problems, is ill posed. For example, the image in figure 3.5a could be produced by more than one 3D object, but we usually perceive only one, a cube. This percept can be "predicted" by imposing "a priori constraints" on the family of possible interpretations— for example, by assuming that the visual system chooses a 3D shape whose contours are planar, and which is "simple" in the sense of having as many symmetries as possible.

Henceforth, a priori constraints will have a special specific meaning. They represent what the visual system "knows" or "assumes" about the 3D objects "out there." Note that these constraints are assumed to be built into the nature of the perceiving organism, which has been dealing successfully with objects "out there" throughout its evolutionary history. Objects "out there" are not arbitrary collections of points and features in 3D space. Instead, they possess the following permanent characteristics. Objects are always spatially cohesive: An object comes in one piece, rather than in more than one. They are opaque: The back part of an object is not seen. Opaqueness presents a potential problem because not all features of the object are seen. Opaqueness, however, simplifies figure–ground organization (see figure 3.12). Next, objects "out there" are always 3D; they have volume. This means that visual data, such as binocular disparity, are not needed to know that an object has some depth. Many objects, including humans and animals, are symmetrical. Objects also tend to be piecewise rigid. Their parts are rigid but often capable of moving relative to each other.

The importance of a priori constraints such as "good figure" and "simplicity" in visual perception was emphasized by the Gestalt psychologists (see chapter 1). The Gestalt psychologists made much of the fact that a circle was the simplest of all possible 2D figures because its contour enclosed the largest possible surface area.[16] It was also aesthetically pleasing because a circle is the most symmetrical of all possible 2D shapes. Note that simplicity of a circle can be captured by a single measure called "compactness," which is the ratio of the surface area A to the square of its perimeter P.

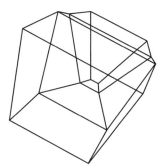 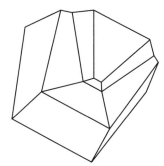

Figure 3.12
A transparent polyhedron is more difficult to see than an opaque one.

This ratio is maximal for a circle. For the 3D case involving a sphere, Gestalt psychologists even offered a physical model, a soap bubble. Here, a sphere is the simplest 3D shape because for a given surface area S, its volume V is maximal (Koffka, 1935, p. 107). The soap bubble "determines" this shape automatically by means of surface tension. However, very few of these Gestalt concepts can be described so simply. In particular, neither Gestalt psychologists themselves nor their successors during the Cognitive Revolution succeeded in showing how the simplicity principle can be applied to objects other than cubes or spheres. Regularization theory can provide a systematic method for doing it.

The application of regularization theory is illustrated on a simple example shown in figure 3.13. Figure 3.13a shows a circle. We see a continuous line with a perfectly symmetrical (simple) shape despite the fact that there are a relatively small number of visual receptors in a given area and they are not arranged regularly. Figure 3.13b and 3.13c illustrate how the visual data would actually look when an observer is presented with a circle. Clearly, the percept is much more like the distal stimulus, a circle, than its retinal image (a set of discrete points). How is this accomplished? Assume first that the visual system "knows" that figure 3.13c was produced by the simplest shape, a circle. In such a case, visual reconstruction of the circle calls for nothing more than a regression analysis. Specifically, the task would be to find the diameter and the coordinates of the center of a circle that provides the best least-squares fit to the retinal data points. However, if the visual system does not "know" that the retinal image was produced by a circle, the analysis must be more sophisticated than a regression. There

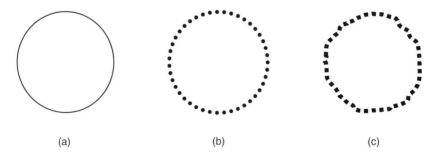

(a)   (b)   (c)

Figure 3.13
Distal stimulus—a circle (a). Due to the discrete nature of retinal sampling, the visual system receives the visual data in a form like that in (b) or even (c).

is good reason to assume that the visual system "regularizes" this problem by doing two things: (i) looking for a "closed" curve that is "smooth" everywhere and (ii) fitting the data points well (think about the Gestalt perceptual organizing principles called "closure" and "good continuation" here). Obviously, the two requirements, namely, fitting data and, at the same time, producing a simple percept, may conflict with each other. This conflict must be resolved by deciding the relative importance that should be given to simplicity and fitting data. Regularization theory provides a method for resolving this conflict. In regularization theory, this is done by using what is called a "cost function," which is the weighted combination of the two requirements (see appendix C, section C.12, for mathematical details and appendix C, section C.13, for probabilistic formulation of regularization). Here, the veridical percept, that is, perceiving a continuous, closed circular curve, corresponds to finding the unique minimum of the cost function.

Regularization theory works even better with 3D shapes. The role of the simplicity principle in the perception of 3D shapes did not receive much attention from the original Gestalt psychologists but was studied systematically by those who revived the Gestalt approach during the Cognitive Revolution between 1950 and 1980. These cognitive psychologists showed that simplicity played a role in determining (i) whether a line drawing is perceived as a 2D or 3D shape (Hochberg & McAlister, 1953), (ii) the veridicality of the perception of the 3D orientations of the edges of a box (Attneave & Frost, 1969), and (iii) the veridicality of the perception of simple 3D shapes (Perkins, 1972, 1976). They were not, however, able to provide a general definition of what they meant by "simplicity" or to include this concept in some kind of a computational model. Poggio et al.'s (1985) approach makes it possible, but they confined their work to developing Marr's 2.5D model (appendix C, section C.14, gives three examples). They did not do any work on shape itself. The application of the inverse problems framework to the study of shape will be presented in the last section of chapter 4 and in chapter 5.

3.5 The Role of Figure–Ground Organization

The same year Poggio et al. (1985) published their paper on the application of regularization theory in vision there was another development that tried to remedy problems inherent in Marr's paradigm. This time, rather than trying to modify Marr's use of a 2.5D sketch, the emphasis was put on the role of figure–ground organization, the fundamental aspect of human vision that was left out of Marr's theory. This new development started with Lowe (1985), who used three rules of perceptual organization in 3D shape recognition. He tried to solve the 3D shape recognition problem, as defined by Roberts (1965), but with two modifications. First, Lowe developed an algorithm that was able to recognize smooth objects, not only polyhedra. Second, Lowe used a perspective, rather than projective transformation. Lowe's algorithm started with finding and grouping edges by using proximity, collinearity, and parallelism. After contours representing a single object were grouped, they were used to perform shape matching. Lowe's algorithm only worked for a small set of predefined objects. Its scope was quite limited, but the book in which he described his research led to a series of papers on machine implementation of Gestalt rules of perceptual organization. Some of them concentrated on the grouping principles themselves (Guy & Medioni, 1996; Alter & Basri, 1998). Others tried to relate grouping to subsequent shape reconstruction and recognition (Malik & Maydan, 1989; Kim & Nevatia, 1999). This interest led to a series of workshops on perceptual organization in computer vision (e.g., Boyer & Sarkar, 2000) as well as special issues of computer vision journals (e.g., Boyer & Sarkar, 1999). Very little progress was made, however, because figure–ground organization is a difficult computational problem. Solving it is equivalent to finding a global minimum of a cost function. Global optimization is computationally intractable. It is known, however, that the human visual system establishes figure–ground organization reliably, quickly, and accurately. This achievement encouraged both machine and human vision scientists to try explain how this could be done. The fact that the human visual system can do it so well suggested that this global optimization task can be solved (approximately) without performing global search. The class of algorithms that can do this is called "pyramid algorithms." Despite their potential, to date, pyramid algorithms have been applied primarily to perceptual grouping problems not directly related to 3D shape reconstruction (Jolion & Rosenfeld, 1994; Jolion & Kropatsch, 1998).

This effort within the machine vision community was of special importance because it encouraged developing computational models of figure–

ground organization. It also revived interest in figure–ground organization within the human vision community. These developments contributed importantly to developing a new paradigm for studying reconstruction of 3D shape. This work made it clear that a priori constraints are critical in achieving figure–ground organization. The realization that a priori constraints were needed to handle figure–ground organization called attention to the fact that they will surely also be needed to reconstruct the 3D shape of an object from its 2D image on the retina.

To summarize, the machine vision community did not solve the "big problem" of shape perception. Most members of this community, following Marr's (1982) lead, assumed that solving the problem inherent in the 2.5D sketch would, in itself, take care of shape. One way of thinking of this is to realize that these workers were committed to a "taking slant into account" explanation of this unique perceptual property. Despite this unfortunate commitment, the machine vision community did accomplish a number of things that prepared the way for progress. First, the machine vision community provided both a mathematical and a computational treatment of the geometry involved in image formation in both calibrated and uncalibrated cameras. Specifically, they formulated, and proved, the necessary and sufficient conditions for the uniqueness of the image-understanding problem. Second, the machine vision community introduced the concepts of, and provided formalisms for, (i) new types of invariants (perspective and model-based) and (ii) solution of inverse problems. Finally, this community took an active role in reviving the Gestalt ideas related to figure–ground organization. This community, however, did not take these tools as far as it could have, probably because it did not appreciate the *uniqueness* of shape in visual perception. They, like all of their predecessors, dealt with shape as a derivative (or secondary) rather than as a primary perceptual feature.

4   Formalisms Enter into the Study of Shape Perception

Research on human shape perception during the last twenty-five years was "shaped" to a large degree by concepts and formalisms provided by the machine vision community. Psychophysical research during this period was dominated by Marr's paradigm. The neo-Gestalt approach to shape, adopted after the Cognitive Revolution, was largely abandoned during this period. Marr's paradigm dominated psychophysical research because it was timely. It coincided with the invention and perfection of computer graphics software and hardware, including virtual reality systems. It encouraged researchers to study the role of depth cues (texture, shading, motion, and binocular disparity) in shape perception because individual depth cues could be easily manipulated. Furthermore, these computer-generated stimuli were more realistic, a development that satisfied the expectations of those who were trained in either the Gibsonian or the Brunswikian tradition (Gibson, 1950, 1966; Brunswik, 1956). Recall that Gibson and Marr, two of the most influential people in vision research between 1950 and 1980, despite many differences, agreed on (i) the importance of the surfaces of objects and (ii) the irrelevance of figure–ground organization in shape perception. This consensus left students of human shape perception with little alternative but to study surfaces. Gibson died in 1979 and Marr in 1980, but each of them left many very active followers who tried to elaborate the theories of their mentors. Others, who were not members of these cliques, felt that they had to test various elements of these two approaches. This also contributed to their popularity. There were only a handful of researchers who did not study the perception of surfaces during this period. These researchers (e.g., Shepard, Biederman, Farah) did recognize the unique status of shape and began to explore the implications of this important fact.

This chapter describes representative work of both groups following Marr's death. It describes work emerging directly from Marr's paradigm and also work by those who tried to overcome some of the problems with Marr's paradigm that had become apparent by that time.

4.1   Marr's Influence

Marr's paradigm, particularly his concept of the 2.5D sketch, raised a number of questions that could be tested in psychophysical research. The two most important experimental questions were the following: (i) Can information about the orientation of surfaces be used to perceive 3D shapes, and (ii) can information about depth be used to perceive 3D shapes? The main conclusion that can be drawn from *all of these experiments* is that the perceptual representation available in the 2.5D sketch is substantially less reliable than the perceptual representation of the 3D shape itself. This conclusion should encourage the reader to seriously consider accepting the author's claim that Marr's 2.5D sketch cannot be used to explain shape perception (a claim that will be supported in detail later).

4.1.1   Can Information about the Orientation of Surfaces Be Used to Perceive 3D Shapes?

Koenderink and his colleagues performed a systematic series of studies of the perception of 3D surfaces. Representative papers include Koenderink, van Doorn, and Kappers (1992, 1994, 1995, 1996); Koenderink and van Doorn (1995); Koenderink et al. (1997); and Todd et al. (1996).

This series of experiments examined how well humans perceive the 3D orientations of surfaces. These orientations, when expressed in the coordinate system of the observer, constitute Marr's 2.5D sketch. The surfaces in these experiments were viewed either monocularly or binocularly, in the presence or absence of other depth cues, such as shading and texture. The subject adjusted the aspect ratio and the 2D orientation of a probe so that it was perceived as "lying" on the 3D surface. This probe was used to measure the perceived slant and tilt of the surface at a particular point. The experimenter used these judgments of local orientations to reconstruct the surface after collecting surface orientation judgments at many points on the surface. The reconstructed surface was assumed to represent the perceived 3D shape of this surface.

One of the main results reported by Koenderink and his colleagues was that there was considerable variability across their subjects, as well as across their viewing conditions. For each individual subject, tilt was judged quite reliably, but slant was not (Koenderink, van Doorn, & Kappers, 1992). The fact that slant judgments are not reliable was not really news. Stavrianos (1945) had already demonstrated this fact using planar (2D) figures, and her results had been replicated in many other studies (e.g., Perrone, 1980; Stevens, 1983). The fact that tilt judgments are fairly reliable *was* news (see Stevens, 1983, who observed this first). Both of these results provide a test of Marr's theory of shape. According to Marr's theory, perception of shape cannot be more reliable than the perception of its 3D orientation because in Marr's theory, shape is perceived "by taking slant into account." We have known that "taking into account" explanations of shape do not work. This had been shown by Stavrianos (1945) (see chapter 1). Stavrianos showed that reducing the availability of depth cues harmed judgments about slant, but not about the shape of a planar figure. Stavrianos' result was extended by Pizlo (1994), who showed that the slanted 2D shape was perceived reliably when slant was varied unpredictably from trial to trial, but not when tilt was varied unpredictably from trial to trial. If Marr's theory is accepted, then, in light of Koenderink et al.'s results, unpredictable tilt should harm perceived shape less than unpredictable slant because tilt is easier to estimate in the visual stimulus. The fact that unpredictable tilt harms perceived shape more than unpredictable slant strongly suggests that the perception of surfaces uses different mechanisms than are used for the perception of shapes. This conclusion runs counter to Marr's theory.

Recently, Li and Pizlo (2006) performed a much-needed direct test of Marr's theory of shape. An observer was shown a line drawing of a box (parallelepiped) and was asked to make judgments of the 3D orientations of three visible surfaces, as well as of their shapes. Using Marr's terminology, judgments about the orientations of surfaces involve a viewer-centered coordinate system and judgments about the shapes of faces involve an object-centered coordinate system. Note that an image of a parallelepiped almost always leads to the percept of a parallelepiped because a symmetry constraint operates with this kind of shape. Li and Pizlo (2006) used Koenderink et al.'s (1992) elliptical probe to measure the perception of the 3D orientations of the faces of the box. The shape judgments were obtained by asking the observer to adjust the aspect ratio and the angle of each of the three visible faces. For example, when a line drawing was perceived as a cube, the observer adjusted the shape of each of the three faces to be a square. Each of these two types of judgments can be used to reconstruct a 3D shape. The main question was whether these two types of judgments, viewer-centered and object-centered, led to the same 3D reconstructed object. They did not. According to Marr, they should. This result implies that the perceived 3D shape is not derived from the perceived orientations of surfaces. Later, it will be shown that the perceived 3D shape is derived from the application of shape constraints to the 2D shape on the retina.

The interest in surfaces inspired by Marr (1982) continues to figure prominently in psychophysical experiments. Todd and Norman (2003) extended the work of Koenderink and his colleagues from judgments about the 3D orientation of a surface relative to the observer to judgments about the 3D orientation of one surface relative to another. In effect, they tested how well a human observer can judge 3D spatial properties within an object-centered coordinate system, the coordinate system used to represent 3D shape in Marr's theory. In their first experiment, the observers were presented with two textured planes forming a dihedral angle (a corner), and the task was to adjust this angle so that it was perceived as a right (90 deg) angle. Binocular disparity was the only cue that was available to see the angle. Note that the two planes were presented in isolation. There was no 3D object. In other words, the authors tested the "perception of shape" by using a single feature, an angle, *in the absence of any shape*, itself. According to Marr's theory, but only according to Marr's theory, this is an appropriate thing to do. The observers found this task to be very unnatural and difficult. Variability across the observers was large, and their judgments showed large systematic errors. These results should have been expected because it was known that the percept of the 3D orientation of a single surface is quite unreliable. It follows that the percept of a more complex feature, namely, the 3D orientation of one surface relative to another, should be even more unreliable. The situation is different when a shape is present when the observer judges an angle between surfaces. Perkins (1972) showed this using a very similar task. Perkins' observers were shown line drawings of boxes, similar to those used by Li and Pizlo (2006). The observer's task was to judge whether an angle formed by three planes was a right angle (see chapter 2). Performance was very accurate and reliable.

4.1.2   Can Information about Depth Be Used to Perceive 3D Shapes?

A related set of studies, rooted in Marr's paradigm, addressed the issue of the role of binocular disparity in 3D shape perception. Binocular disparity is one of the most, if not the most effective depth cue. Julesz (1960) had demonstrated that binocular disparity, in the absence of any contours, was sufficient to allow the observer to judge 3D spatial relations among points and features. This demonstration was potentially important because it suggested that 3D *geometrical* space might be mapped *directly* to 3D *perceptual* space. If it could be, there might not be any need to deal with 2D shapes in the perspective images on the retinas. If 2D retinal shapes are not necessary, both depth and shape could be perceived veridically from binocular disparity alone.

4.1.2.1 Can Binocular Disparity, by Itself, Yield Veridical Shape Perception?   Mathematically, binocular disparity is sufficient to compute positions of points and features in 3D space (Longuet-Higgins, 1981). Practically, it is not because in the case of real images of real scenes, even tiny errors in measuring the retinal positions of points and features will lead to large errors in the reconstruction of depth. McKee, Levi, and Bowne (1990) and Norman et al. (1996) asked subjects to make judgments about 3D distances when binocular disparity was the main, or even the only, cue carrying the 3D information. They found that observers' judgments about distances in 3D space are very inaccurate.

How about binocular judgments of shape? Johnston (1991) used random-dot stereograms ostensibly to test the role of binocular disparity in shape perception. The observer was shown a cylinder with the line of sight parallel to its cross section. The task was to judge whether the cross section was a circle or an ellipse. All aspects of the stimulus were held constant except depth. Johnston found that the shape was not perceived veridically. At small viewing distances, the elliptical cylinder looked too deep; at large viewing distances, it did not look deep enough. The reader should keep in mind that Johnston's experiment deals with depth perception, not with shape perception, because she used ellipses, the family of shapes that precludes studying shape constancy because it only has one parameter (see discussion of Thouless' experiments in chapter 1).

Johnston's (1991) experiment was replicated a number of times. Sometimes elliptical cylinders were used, but other objects, such as cones, sine wave surfaces, and pyramids, were used as well (e.g., Tittle et al., 1995; Durgin et al., 1995; Glennerster, Rogers, & Bradshaw, 1996; Bradshaw, Parton, & Glennerster, 2000; Todd & Norman, 2003). What was common in all these studies was that depth was the only property used to discriminate among the stimuli. As a result, all of these experiments are relevant *only* to depth perception. They are not relevant to shape perception. How could experiments like these be changed so as to make it possible to use them to find out something about shape? There are two general guidelines: (i) Use structured objects, whose shapes are characterized by more than one or two parameters, and (ii) use more than one viewing orientation of the objects relative to the observer. The second guideline is especially important because it is the only way to study shape constancy. Remember that shape is important primarily because of constancy. It gives objects their identity and potential usefulness. If you want to study shape, rather than some other visual property, you can find out whether you are actually studying shape by including a condition designed to estimate the amount of shape constancy achieved with the particular stimuli you chose to use. All you need to do is to remember to present your stimuli from more than a single viewpoint. Put simply, the best way (certainly the sensible way) to study shape is to study shape constancy and to do this with families of shapes with sufficient complexity to allow constancy to manifest itself. Prototypical examples of experiments that followed these guidelines are Stavrianos (1945), Shepard and Metzler (1971), Biederman and Gerhardstein (1993), and Pizlo and Stevenson (1999). Figure 4.1 shows the kinds of stimuli that should be used in such experiments. Two symmetrical objects are shown. The only difference between them is that one is thicker than the other. It is easy to see that these two shapes are different even though binocular disparity information is entirely absent. Furthermore, each of these simple, meaningless objects is easy to recognize from any viewing direction. Depth information is not needed here because depth is reconstructed from regularities of the objects themselves such as symmetry (Kontsevich, 2002; Vetter & Poggio, 2002; Pizlo, Li, & Steinman, 2006).

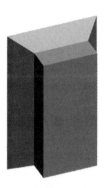 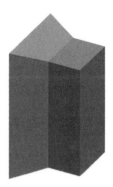

Figure 4.1
These two images could not be produced by the same 3D shape, and they are perceived as different shapes (produced using 3DS Max/Autodesk).

4.1.2.2 Can Binocular Disparity Contribute to Shape Perception? We have seen that binocular disparity in itself cannot lead to veridical shape perception. Can it contribute when other sources of shape information are available?

Several reports have shown that binocular perception of shape is strongly affected by what are called "monocular perspective cues" (Stevens & Brookes, 1988; Stevens, Lees, & Brookes, 1991; van Ee, van Dam, & Erkelens, 2002; Papathomas, 2002). In textbook examples, a monocular perspective cue is usually illustrated by the fact that two or more parallel lines "out there" produce converging lines in a perspective image. More generally, one speaks of a monocular perspective cue when symmetrical shapes "out there" produce images with distorted symmetry. Figure 4.2 shows an example. The distorted symmetry in the 2D perspective image illustrated in this figure provides useful information about the 3D orientation of the object "out there" as well as useful information about the shape of the 3D object itself. Once perspective cues are available, what is the relative potential contribution of binocular disparity?

This was tested by Pizlo, Li, and Francis (2005), who put perspective cues in conflict with binocular disparity. Their main experiment was performed with the stereoscopic images shown in figure 4.3. Both pairs, when fused, lead to the perception of a cube. The stimuli in (b) are identical to those in (a) except that the three edges forming the Y junction have been removed. In the experiment, the images viewed by the left eye were

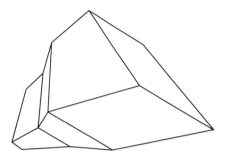

Figure 4.2
Illustration of a monocular perspective cue. This is an image of a mirror-symmetrical object. The image itself is not symmetrical. Its symmetry is distorted.

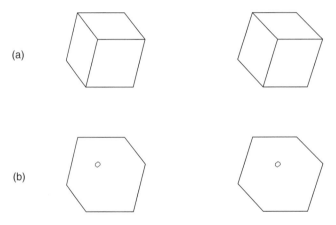

(a)

(b)

Figure 4.3
Stimuli used by Pizlo, Li, and Francis (2005).

stationary, but those viewed by the right eye were not. The cube viewed by the right eye oscillated around the vertical axis (see http://viper.psych .purdue.edu/pizlo_cubes/). When only the right eye was open, a rigid oscillating cube was perceived for both (a) and (b). When both eyes were open, the observer fused the moving and the stationary cubes. According to conventional binocular theory (Julesz, 1971; Regan, 2000), the observer should see a nonrigid cube whose corner at the Y junction moves toward and away from the eye (left) with the stationary cube. This percept was observed in (b), but not in (a). In (a), the observer perceived a rigid cube oscillating from left to right. These results show two important things: (i) The visual system first establishes figure–ground organization, that is, it establishes which contours and regions in the image represent a single 3D object; and (ii) once figure–ground organization has been established, binocular disparity comes into play, but only to determine the spatial relations across different objects—here, between the dot and the outline in (b)—not among parts within a single object—here, among the corners of the cube in (a).[1] The percept in (a) is determined exclusively by perspective cues; binocular disparity is ignored entirely.

This left the question of whether information from multiple cues, such as shading, texture, motion, and binocular disparity, is used to perceive a 3D shape. Prior studies on the perception of *3D surfaces* showed that using information from multiple depth cues is beneficial (e.g., Schrater, & Kersten, 2000; Bülthoff, 1991; Hillis et al., 2004; Landy et al., 1995; Knill & Saunders, 2003; Backus et al., 1999; Doorschot, Kappers, & Koenderink, 2001; Bülthoff & Mallot, 1988). Can information from multiple cues be used to perceive 3D *shapes*? Li and Pizlo (2005) examined this directly in a shape constancy experiment with complex polyhedral shapes (see figure 4.4). They found that 3D shape is perceived reliably even when only the edges of polyhedra are shown; adding shading and texture contributes

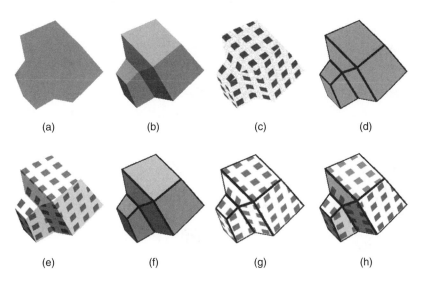

(a)   (b)   (c)   (d)

(e)   (f)   (g)   (h)

Figure 4.4
Stimuli in Li and Pizlo's (2005) experiment. The objects in that experiment were rendered with various combinations of the following cues: shading, texture, edges, and binocular disparity. The binocular disparity cue is not illustrated here.

little, if anything. Adding binocular disparity does improve performance. However, binocular performance is not very good, unless monocular performance is very good, as well. This means that if simplicity constraints, such as symmetry, cannot produce a good 3D shape percept from a single 2D image, binocular disparity contributes nothing! These results strongly suggest that the perceptual mechanisms involved in the binocular perception of 3D shapes are very similar, if not identical, to those involved in the perception of 3D shapes from a single 2D image. This is illustrated in figure 4.5, where two stereoscopic pairs of images are shown. The pair on the top has zero binocular disparity and no shading or texture, and the pair on the bottom has all three depth cues. When fused, the two objects are perceived as having the same 3D shape, although the depth of the one in the bottom is greater (more vivid). Clearly, the perception of depth seems to play a secondary role, at best, in the perception of shape. This is as it should be. In a world in which questions such as "What is that over there?" and "Where is it?" are commonplace, the perception of shape, depth, and direction would be best served by having three relatively independent mechanisms. All of the available evidence to date points to the fact that depth, direction, and shape function independently.

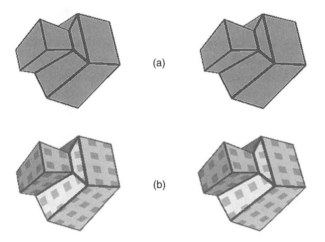

(a)

(b)

Figure 4.5
Stereoscopic stimuli (crossed fusion): (a) edges and no disparity; (b) edges, shading, texture, and binocular disparity (viewing distance twelve times larger than the distance between the stimuli within a pair).

4.2   If Depth Does Not Contribute to the 3D Shape Percept, What Does? (Poggio's Influence)

How is the three-dimensionality of a shape percept produced from a 2D retinal image? How is the 3D shape percept produced, if not by taking depth into account? There must be another mechanism. Poggio, Torre, and Koch (1985) prepared the way for answering this question when they introduced the inverse problem and regularization theory into vision science (see chapter 3). It is assumed in this framework that the visual system uses a priori information about the objects "out there" to constrain the family of possible 3D percepts. This approach provides a way to produce a unique as well as a veridical 3D percept. A substantial number of papers providing mathematical and computational tools to describe the joint effect of the 2D retinal image and a priori constraints have been published since Poggio et al.'s influential paper (e.g., Clark & Yuille, 1990; Knill & Richards, 1996; Kersten, Mamassian, & Yuille, 2004). As indicated in chapter 3, Poggio, and those he influenced, were concerned with the perception of the third dimension in the 2.5D sketch. As a result, the a priori constraints they used were designed to produce 3D *surfaces*, not 3D *shapes*. Furthermore, their concern was directed primarily toward formulating computational models rather than toward verifying their models with psychophysical tests. There were only a handful of studies that actually tested these models. The three most recent studies, namely, Knill (1992), Saunders and Knill (2001), and Mamassian and Landy (1998), will be described next.

Knill (1992) tested the role of a geodesic constraint. This constraint says that the curvature of a surface's contours represents the curvature of the surface itself (Hilbert & Cohn-Vossen, 1952). This constraint reduces the family of possible 3D surfaces and, under some additional assumptions, allows a unique reconstruction of the surface (Stevens, 1981, 1986). Knill presented the observer with a 3D corrugated surface produced by shading and a superimposed patch. The contours of the patch were either straight-line segments, which are geodesics on a planar surface, or wavy lines that were geodesics of the corrugated surface. If a geodesic constraint is involved in the perception of 3D surfaces, the observer should be able to classify the patches into two categories: Either a patch is a planar transparent patch "floating" in front of the surface or it is a part of the surface itself. The observers were able to classify the patches in this manner. In his second experiment, Knill showed that observers were able to perceive 3D surfaces even when the surface contours were not exactly geodesic lines. In other words, the visual system is robust in the sense that it can reconstruct the surface even when the assumption about the geodesic lines is not satisfied exactly. In a more recent paper, Saunders and Knill (2001) tested the role of a symmetry constraint in binocular perception of the 3D orientation of planar (2D) shapes and showed that this constraint systematically affects monocular and binocular percepts. When binocular disparity conflicted with the symmetry constraint, these two were combined to produce the 3D percept.

Finally, consider Mamassian and Landy's (1998) report of a study in which the observers were presented with two curves forming an X and were asked to classify the contours as being either elliptical (egg-shaped) or hyperbolic (saddle-shaped). The subject's responses were then explained by a Bayesian model, which used three constraints: (i) The surfaces are convex, (ii) they are viewed from above, and (iii) the surface contours are lines of curvature that are geodesic lines.

To summarize, during the last 20 years, a growing body of evidence suggested that constraints could play a role in perception of 3D *surfaces*. This work, however, did not go beyond Marr's paradigm. It did not deal with the perception of 3D *shapes*. It only dealt with *surfaces*. This work, however, did set the stage for studying the role of constraints in the perception of 3D shapes.

4.3   The Uniqueness of Shape Is Finally Recognized

4.3.1   Mental Rotation of 3D Shapes

Shepard and Metzler's (1971) research initiated the modern interest in the 3D perceptual representation of objects (see Shepard & Cooper, 1982, for a review of research that became sufficiently popular for it to be called a cottage industry). Shepard and Metzler made their contribution to shape perception indirectly. They were primarily interested in higher level cognitive processes, rather than the perception of 3D objects from 2D images. They worked in parallel with Marr and were not influenced by his commitment to the 2.5D sketch. They were well aware of the contributions of the neo-Gestalt psychologists who were studying perception of 3D objects from 2D images (Hochberg & McAlister, 1953; Attneave & Frost, 1969; Perkins, 1972), so it is not surprising that they used perspective 2D drawings of structured 3D objects to test their subjects' ability to rotate objects mentally. They were under no pressure to worry about the basis on which their 2D images could produce compelling 3D percepts. They also saw no reason for using depth cues, as individuals influenced by Marr felt compelled to include in their experiments. The effectiveness of their 2D stimuli in producing vivid 3D shape percepts, and the notoriety of their result, called attention to the possibility of using stimuli like theirs for research on the perception of shape itself. An example of their stimuli is shown in figure 4.6. Each object consisted of three or four rectangular bars forming two or three Ls. The subject was shown two such objects, each having a different 3D orientation, and was asked to judge whether the objects were identical, except for their orientations. When the objects were not identical, one of the Ls in one object was a mirror image of the corresponding L in the other object. In this case, one of the objects could not be transformed into the other by rigid motion. Shepard and Metzler wanted to find out whether the subjects rotated the objects mentally when they did this task. They assumed that mental rotation would take time, and the amount of time it took would be proportional to the angle required to rotate one object to match the orientation of the other. The subjects' reaction times varied systematically, allowing the authors to conclude that their subjects were actually rotating the perceived 3D representations of objects mentally. This experiment, which was designed to study higher

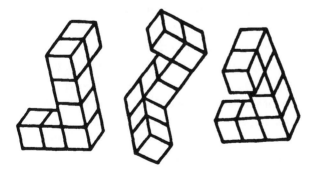

Figure 4.6
An example of the objects used by Shepard and Metzler (1971) (From Shepard & Cooper, 1982, MIT Press).

mental processes, is also important for the study of shape perception. The fact that a 3D shape can be rotated mentally, which simulates the conditions where an observer walks around an object, or the object is rotated in front of the observer, is analogous to the conditions present in shape constancy experiments. Shepard and Metzler's (1971) 2D stimuli produced a "veridical 3D percept" of an object "out there" that had *no features other than its shape* to reveal its identity! The fact that a 2D image could produce a 3D percept of shape and that this percept is not affected by the viewing orientation paved the way for Biederman's (1985) recognition-by-components theory of shape perception.

4.3.2   Shape Recognition by Components

4.3.2.1   Biederman's (1985) Theory   Biederman's theory quickly became the center of attention in both the human and machine vision communities. Biederman, unlike most others interested in shape, was unusual because he was familiar with all of the important milestones in the history of shape perception in both communities. He reviewed all of the important work in his seminal paper and made a serious attempt to synthesize all of the existing knowledge about shape available in 1985. Biederman attempted to (i) explain the perception of arbitrary 3D shapes; (ii) account for errors and reaction times observed during both recognition and reconstruction experiments on 3D shape; (iii) provide sufficient technical details to make it possible to implement his theory with computer simulations, as well as to test it in psychophysical experiments with human subjects; and (iv) relate the perception of 3D shapes to other fundamental aspects of vision, such as figure–ground organization and the Gestalt simplicity principle.

Biederman called his theory of shape reconstruction "recognition-by-components" (RBC), an acronym that captured the essence of his underlying idea. According to Biederman, an arbitrary 3D shape can be represented as an arrangement of several simple parts he called "geons." Geons resemble boxes, cones, spheres, and cylinders. In RBC theory, objects differ with respect to the particular geons that make them up and how they are arranged. Biederman himself considered his theory as analogous to spoken language, primarily because both are composed of a limited number of simple elements, phonemes for language and geons for shape. The analogy between shape and language perception had been around for more than a decade (Hoffman & Richards, 1984; Huffman, 1971; Minsky, 1975), but Biederman was the first to formulate, and test, a theory of human shape perception based on it.

Biederman, unlike Marr and Gibson, assumed that figure–ground organization *is* critical in 3D shape perception. Specifically, he postulated that the retinal (or camera) image has sufficient information to allow identification (recognition) of geons. For example, a retinal image of a cube is quite different from a retinal image of a circular cone. One should be able to recognize 3D parts of an arbitrary object by identifying straight and curved lines, groups of parallel lines and curves, and patterns of mirror symmetry, as well as junctions of contours. It follows that *3D shape* can be recognized on the basis of the information contained in the *2D shape* of its retinal image.

Biederman emphasized the fact that the recognition of 3D shape depends on the recognition of the geons making it up and their 3D spatial arrangement. With this emphasis, Biederman effectively adopted an "atomistic" position by claiming that the whole shape is produced by adding up its parts. Many 3D objects have parts, so it is not surprising that many objects can be recognized by recognizing their parts. This does *not* mean, however, that the perceived 3D shape of an object is *the sum of the perceived shapes of its parts*. The 3D shapes of the parts, as well as the 3D shape of the object, could be just as easily recognized from their 2D shapes by applying simplicity constraints. For example, if a 3D object, which is composed of several parts, is symmetrical, its 2D retinal image will be approximately symmetrical. By using a symmetry constraint, the 3D shape can be derived without recognizing *any of its parts*. Note that when Biederman adopted his "atomistic" position, which he claimed was rooted in the Gestalt simplicity principle, he actually had developed a theory that would have been anathema to the Gestalt psychologists because it violated one of their fundamental assumptions, namely, von Ehrenfel's canon that the "*Gestaltqualität* [form quality or shape] is different from the sum of its parts." What encouraged Biederman to adopt an "atomistic" approach to shape perception? Biederman knew that one of the main obstacles in making machines "see" was their inability to recognize partially occluded objects in natural environments. Humans, unlike machines, do this very well. Biederman assumed that humans' ability to recognize partially occluded objects derives from humans' ability to recognize parts of objects, which are not occluded.

Although this assumption seems reasonable, it does not justify ignoring the shape of the entire 3D object. In real images of real scenes, the information about a single isolated part of an object is often less reliable than the information about the whole shape. One should do better by using all the information available than by using only part of it. Biederman's theory inspired a good deal of research by a number of people, despite the obvious shortcomings just described. It was the first theory to directly address the important problem of how the percept of a 3D shape is derived from the 2D shape of its retinal image. Both reasons warrant discussing Biederman's RBC theory in some depth.

Biederman proposed that as few as thirty-six geons would be sufficient to model the universe of 3D shapes. This number was derived, somewhat arbitrarily, by considering all possible combinations of basic geometric features, such as junctions, symmetries, and curvatures of parts of contours that could be used to characterize the larger class of objects, known as "generalized cones" (also known as "generalized cylinders" or "sweeps"). Biederman's contribution consisted of dramatically reducing the set of infinitely many generalized cones that were described by Binford (1971). Binford (1971) himself was not concerned with restricting the number of 3D shapes that would be used (Biederman's requirement) but rather with restricting the number of parameters required to represent infinitely many smooth 3D shapes for machine vision applications. In 1971, when Binford published, the machine vision community only knew how to handle polyhedra, so Binford made a very useful contribution. If computational models of vision were to be general models, they had to be able to deal with more than polyhedra. Dealing with arbitrarily smooth surfaces requires many parameters. In the extreme case, the number of parameters would be infinitely large, as large as the number of points on a surface. Binford's generalized cones offered a way to simplify the representation of smooth surfaces. Binford's approach showed how a fairly small set of parameters could be used to generate and represent a quite large family of 3D parts. Figure 4.7 shows several examples of generalized cones used in machine vision applications.[2]

There is an additional advantage of using RBC theory. If parts of a complex object can be recognized from any viewing direction, shape constancy may be easy to achieve. It follows that determining the extent to which shape constancy is achieved is a natural way to test RBC theory.

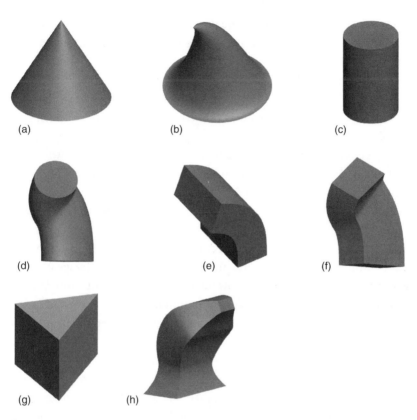

Figure 4.7
Examples of generalized cones. The shape of the cross section is constant in each, and the eccentricity angle is 90 deg. The axis is straight in (a), (c), and (g). The axis is curved and planar in (b), (e), and (h) (produced using 3DS Max/Autodesk).

Shape constancy experiments before Biederman used mostly simple 2D shapes that were geometrically, rather than qualitatively, different from one another (e.g., ellipses with different aspect ratios). They mainly asked questions about the viewing conditions under which shape constancy fails. Biederman changed all that by using solid objects composed of qualitatively different parts. In this kind of experiment, humans could, and did, achieve shape constancy reliably. Reaction times were short, and they did not depend on the 3D orientation of the object, suggesting that mental rotation was not involved. Finally, the proportion of correct judgments was high, even with exposure durations as short as 100 ms (Biederman, 1987; Biederman & Gerhardstein, 1993). Such fine performance can be explained by assuming that only qualitative features of shapes were utilized in his shape constancy experiments. The reliable analysis of quantitative features would require considerably more time.[3]

To summarize, Biederman's (1985) RBC theory forced visionists to change the way they thought about 3D shape perception, but the theory itself did not lead to computational models that could be applied to real images of real objects. No one to date has succeeded in providing an algorithm for finding geons in real images. Biederman assumed that this task would not be difficult. He may have been influenced by Gibson and thought that geons can be "picked up" from the 2D image directly, and that they would "pop out" like the special features in one of Treisman and Gelade's (1980) displays. They did not, so it is now commonly acknowledged that the visual system must perform an effective figure–ground organization, one that identifies the contour representing (belonging to) the image of a particular 3D shape. Biederman was aware of the importance of figure–ground organization, but he kept its role to a minimum in his theory. This was a mistake. The importance of figure–ground organization can not be minimal in a successful computational model of shape.

4.3.2.2 Pentland's (1986) Component Theory of Shape Perception   Pentland (1986) published a very similar theory at about the same time as Biederman (Biederman's paper was submitted in July 1985, Pentland's in August 1985). Both Biederman and Pentland were stimulated by the computational research on generalized cones as candidates for modeling parts of complex objects (Binford, 1971; Marr & Nishihara, 1978; Marr, 1982). They both decided to restrict the family of shape parts by using symmetry, but their parts were different. Biederman's parts were generalized cones, while Pentland's were superquadrics.

Pentland proposed a set of fifty-six superquadrics, which were simple 3D shapes, such as boxes, spheres, cylinders, and cones. These shapes were characterized by a small set of parameters. By using parameterized shapes, he was able to produce infinitely many 3D shapes belonging to the fifty-six families. As a result, the parts used by Pentland were able to describe more closely real 3D shapes than Biederman could with his geons. However, Pentland did not go beyond the stage of describing the parts of objects. Biederman used the parts not only to describe but also to recognize shapes from their parts. Dickinson built on both, by (i) elaborating Biederman's theory and (ii) incorporating Pentland's emphasis on parametric modeling with the use of superquadrics.

4.3.2.3 Dickinson's Elaboration of Biederman's and Pentland's Theories

Biederman's (1985) paper had an immediate impact on the computer vision community. However, all attempts to develop computational models for geon reconstruction and recognition based on Biederman's RBC theory led to systems that were geon specific (e.g., Bergevin & Levine, 1992a, b, 1993; Jacot-Descombes & Pun, 1992; Munck-Fairwood, 1991; Munck-Fairwood & Barreau, 1991; Du & Munck-Fairwood 1993, 1995; Eklundh & Olofsson, 1992; Hummel et al., 1988; Raja & Jain, 1992, 1994; Wu & Levine, 1994; Borges & Fisher, 1997). These models failed to become a commonly accepted approach in computer vision for two reasons (Dickinson, Bergevin, Biederman, Eklundh, Jain, Munck-Fairwood & Pentland, 1997): (i) Many saw Biederman's choice of qualitative shape properties defining geons as arbitrary; a different choice of qualitative properties would yield a different set of shape parts, for which the geon reconstruction algorithms would be unsuitable; and (ii) the proposed reconstruction models had only been demonstrated on idealized scenes, where salient contours mapped directly to definitive geon features. In other words, the use of these models was restricted to cases where figure–ground organization had already been established.

Dickinson, Pentland, and Rosenfeld addressed the first problem by developing a more general framework for reconstructing 3D parts that did not depend on geons as the modeling primitives (Dickinson, Pentland, & Rosenfeld, 1990, 1992a, b; Dickinson, Metaxas, & Pentland, 1997). They proposed an object modeling/recognition framework that used 2D views to model a finite set of 3D parts. Unlike traditional aspect graph approaches of the period, which modeled entire objects and where the number of aspects grew both with object complexity and with the number of parts, this framework's database of views was fixed, and dependent only on the size of the part "vocabulary" (e.g., Koenderink & van Doorn, 1979; Ikeuchi & Kanade, 1988; Chakravarty & Freeman, 1982; Kriegman & Ponce, 1990; Plantinga & Dyer, 1990; Sallam & Bowyer, 1991; Shimshoni & Ponce, 1993; Stewman & Bowyer, 1990; Eggert et al., 1993; Eggert & Bowyer, 1990). The part-based views were organized into an *aspect hierarchy*, consisting of topological collections of regions, the component regions, and the component contours of regions. This hierarchy represented the main features of figure–ground organization. Shape parts were considered independent during part reconstruction, and the reconstructed volumes were combined to form a viewpoint-invariant representation (qualitative 3D part configuration) that could serve for fast shape recognition.

The second problem, 3D shape reconstruction from real images of real objects, has remained elusive. The part-based approach led to correct recognitions only in the case of simple images, representing a single 3D object composed of a few parts, like that in figure 4.8a (Dickinson et al., 1992b). This problem emerged because real images do not allow unambiguous

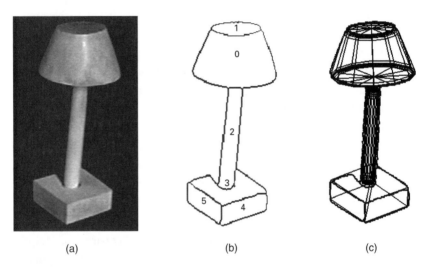

(a)   (b)   (c)

Figure 4.8
(a) Image of a lamp; (b) reconstructed parts of the object by means of Dickinson et al.'s (1992b) OPTICA system. Regions 0 and 1 were correctly grouped into a part-based aspect representing the canonical view of a truncated cone volume; region 2 was not grouped with other regions but was correctly interpreted as an occluded, cylindrical volumetric part; and regions 3, 4, and 5 were correctly grouped into a rectangular volumetric block. Although other interpretations of these regions were computed by the system—for example, region 1 as an ellipsoid volume occluding the top of the truncated cone or region 2 as a bent cylindrical part—such interpretations were assigned lower probabilities. (c) Lamp reconstructed by means of fitting deformable superquadrics to the recovered qualitative shapes shown in (b). The qualitative identities of the parts and their orientations, along with a specification of which contours should be used to identify the parts, all provide strong constraints on the fitting process (with kind permission of the author and the publisher).

recognition of parts. In an effort to work with more realistic objects, the machine vision community steadily migrated toward multiple-view models, in which a 3D shape was represented by a large number of 2D images. Attempts to reconstruct 3D parts from an image are now uncommon. Today's systems focus on 2D configurations of local, image-based features rather than on 3D configurations of shape-based volumetric features.

An approach to 3D shape recognition, based on Pentland's superquadrics, was somewhat more successful. Reconstruction of 3D shapes from image contours is inherently unconstrained, but Dickinson and Metaxas (1994) were able to partially overcome this problem by using qualitative shape models to identify parts and then using the part's identity and the 2D image contours to constrain the fitting of a deformable 3D superquadric to the image data. An illustration of such a reconstruction in the case of a simple 3D object is shown in figure 4.8c. One interesting aspect of Dickinson and Metaxas' shape reconstruction process was that the fitting process was sequential. The parameters of the superquadric were estimated one at a time, leading to a succession of simple optimization problems. The ordering of the parameters in this process was specified manually. Developing an automatic ordering remains an interesting research problem.

To summarize, the theories of Biederman (1985), Pentland (1986), and Dickinson and his colleagues stimulated research in machine vision by putting emphasis on those aspects of 3D shape that make it special, clearly different from other spatial properties such as depth or size. They did this by (i) incorporating simplicity by choosing a small number of simple 3D shapes to recognize and reconstruct natural objects, (ii) ignoring the 2.5D sketch, and (iii) using 3D representations of 3D shapes. Note that simplicity was used in these theories as an *implicit* constraint. That is, these theories assumed that objects have simple shapes. It will be argued in the next chapter that simplicity should be used as an *explicit* constraint. Note also that shape constancy became an important consideration in all of these theories, clearly an important step forward.

4.3.3   Viewpoint Dependence in Shape Perception
Realize that when Biederman showed that human beings demonstrate considerable shape constancy, he did this with 2D line drawings of 3D objects. This was a major event in our understanding of shape perception

because it showed that shape constancy did not require taking depth or slant into account, the belief that had held back research in this area for a very long time. Marr (1982), who had been so influential in vision science, also recognized that human beings showed shape constancy, but he ascribed this critical accomplishment to taking depth and slant into account. This, of course, put Biederman in conflict with Marr (1982), whose position was generally accepted in both human and machine vision communities. As one might expect, Marr's followers, when faced with this difficulty, tried to show that Biederman's results depended on his particular choices of stimuli and that they would not generalize to other stimuli. They only partially succeeded. In particular, they tried to show that the human ability to recognize the shape of a 3D object depends on the orientation of the object relative to the observer. They generated psychophysical data showing that both the proportion of correct responses and reaction time were strongly affected by the viewing orientation of the 3D object relative to the observer. They called this kind of dependence "viewpoint dependence." Note, however, that viewpoint dependence is not necessarily inconsistent with Biederman's theory. Biederman thought that his RBC theory must lead to viewpoint *independence* because the representation of 3D geons is viewpoint independent, but a *viewpoint-independent representation of 3D shape does not imply viewpoint-independent performance*. In other words, computation of invariants need not itself be invariant (Pizlo, 1994; Wagemans et al., 1996; Stankiewicz, 2002). By insisting that performance must be viewpoint independent, Biederman unnecessarily opened his theory to this criticism, and as one might expect, Marr's champions took advantage of Biederman's mistake. The reader should realize that the only way to verify whether the RBC theory predicts viewpoint-independent performance is to implement the theory in the form of a computational model and test it with real images. This has not been done, yet. Had such computational tests been performed, it is very likely that performance would have been viewpoint dependent simply because viewing direction affects the ease with which a shape can be reconstructed.

To summarize, the difficulties associated with formulating theories of shape perception that used Biederman's parts or Marr's 2.5D sketch led researchers to formulate a new approach that would not suffer from the weaknesses inherent in both. These researchers began by examining a feature common to both theories, namely, the emphasis on the three-dimensionality of the percept. They wondered whether removing the assumption that the percept of a 3D object is also 3D would produce a better theory of human shape perception. This new kind of theory claimed, as Helmholtz had 150 years earlier, that the perception of 3D shapes is based on memorizing a large number of 2D views. The modern formulation of this empiristic theory was motivated, at least to some extent, by the psychophysical results on viewpoint dependence. It seemed natural to claim that if shape perception is viewpoint dependent, the perceptual representation of shape itself is based on a number of different 2D views. Tarr was among the first to study the viewpoint dependence systematically. He started with a theory in which 3D shape is represented by *multiple views*, each view being equivalent to a 2.5D representation. Shape constancy in this theory was achieved by means of mental rotation of these 3D shapes (Tarr & Pinker, 1991). Tarr went on to adopt a theory developed by Poggio and Edelman (1990), according to which multiple views refer primarily (or exclusively) to 2D, rather than 2.5D, images. In this theory, shape constancy is achieved by evaluating the similarity among these 2D images rather than by rotating 3D shapes mentally (Tarr et al., 1997, 1998; Hayward & Tarr, 1997). In these experiments, viewpoint dependence was found to be especially strong when unstructured objects, such as polygonal lines, were used. In fact, the multiple view theory of Poggio and Edelman (1990) was developed to account for human performance with such stimuli. This theory obtained additional support from experiments that included other unstructured objects such as spheres with multiples spikes radiating from their surfaces (Edelman & Bülthoff, 1992; Bülthoff & Edelman, 1992). Edelman and Bülthoff, like Rock and DiVita (1987), failed to obtain shape constancy with these objects. The failure to achieve shape constancy with these unstructured stimuli *was to be expected* because 2D images of unstructured stimuli do not convey any useful information about their 3D shape. Some "shape constancy" can be obtained with such unstructured stimuli, but only after observers have been given an extended opportunity to memorize the 2D views.

Can anything else about shape constancy be learned by using unstructured objects as stimuli? Farah, Rochlin, and Klein (1994) performed a series of experiments showing that wire objects are useful, but only when they are studied together with other objects that do lead to shape constancy. They used two classes of stimuli. One consisted of wire objects, whose contours were closed. They did not include a visible surface. The other class of objects had identical contours, but they also had a visible surface. These objects looked like natural potato chips. The subject was shown two objects from one or the other class and was asked to decide whether they had identical shapes. The orientation of the objects relative to the observer was varied, so their retinal images were usually different. If shape constancy was achieved, the subject would be able to identify identical objects regardless of their orientation. Farah et al. (1994) found that performance with wire-only objects was very poor. Performance with "potato chips" was much better. They suggested that the "regularity" and "redundancy" of the surfaces, concepts very close to "simplicity" and "symmetry," might have been the critical factor. They did not develop this idea, but it is worth keeping it in mind because it will be shown later that a new simplicity principle, containing symmetry and two additional constraints, is the critical element in shape perception.

Wire objects were also used by Liu, Knill, and Kersten (1995) and Liu and Kersten (1998). Like Farah et al. (1994), they used wire objects, but not to demonstrate the limits of shape constancy. They used them to demonstrate the role of simplicity (symmetry and planarity) in 3D shape constancy. Specifically, they used four types of objects. Some were symmetrical and planar, and others were not. The subject was first familiarized with eleven views of each object and then tested with either familiar (learned) views of these objects or with a novel, randomly generated view. Performance in shape identification, with both familiar and novel views, was best for stimuli that were symmetrical and planar.

Next, the authors applied an "ideal observer" analysis to their data (Kersten, 1990; Tjan & Legge, 1998). An ideal observer analysis computes the performance of a hypothetical observer who does not have any limitations arising from the ways the human visual system represents, stores, and analyzes the stimuli. In other words, an ideal observer generates the best possible performance given the particular type of input. The authors formulated three types of ideal observers. The first (called 2D Euclidean) assumed that the visual data are represented in the visual system by 2D images. No 3D representation was used. Shape recognition was performed by comparing a given 2D image to the set of stored (memorized) 2D images of objects. To make this "ideal" insensitive to rotations around the line of sight, identification performance was based on many 2D orientations of the test image (Liu et al., 1995). This "ideal" represents a class of multiple-views models of shape like Poggio and Edelman's (1990). The second "ideal" (called 2D affine) was identical to the first, except that it was invariant not only to 2D rotations but also to 2D affine transformations. Finally, the third "ideal" (called 3D) assumed that there are 3D models of shapes in the observer's memory and recognition is performed by verifying whether a given 2D image could have been produced by any of the memorized 3D models. This "ideal" represents a class of models for 3D shape recognition like those of Basri and Ullman (1993), Lowe (1985), and Pizlo and Loubier (2000).

Liu and his colleagues showed, as expected, that human performance was lower than that of the "3D ideal." This was expected because the 3D ideal used 3D representation of shapes but, unlike human observers, did not have any "perceptual" or "memory" noise. They showed next that human performance with novel views of symmetrical and planar stimuli was higher than the 2D Euclidean ideal observer's. This result implies that multiple-views models (such as Poggio & Edelman's, 1990) are not good models of human shape perception. Finally, performance of the 2D affine ideal observer was higher than the humans', but human performance was relatively higher on novel views than on familiar (learned) views. These results, taken together, especially those involving the 2D ideals, clearly show that the human visual system uses 3D representations of 3D shapes (see Stankiewicz, 2002, for a similar conclusion based on different stimuli).

It follows from the studies of Farah et al. (1994) and of Liu and his colleagues that unstructured objects can be used in shape constancy studies, but only as a control condition, when the role of simplicity in 3D shape perception is under study.

4.3.4 The Role of Shape Constraints in Shape Constancy

The experiments that will be described next were based on the assumption that perceived 3D shape depends on the operation of a priori constraints. An alternative basis for achieving shape constancy is needed now that we know that neither the perception of depth nor the memorization of images of objects can do the job. Only a priori constraints can do the job. When this fact became apparent, two types of spatial constraints were available, one of which was local, the other global. Poggio et al. (1985) and those influenced by them, used the following local constraints: smoothness of surfaces and contours, convexity of a surface, and local straightness of surface contours. These constraints are spatially "local" in the sense that they operate on only a small part of a surface at a time. Such constraints proved to be useful only in reconstructing surfaces, not 3D shapes. Bieder-man (1985), Pentland (1986), Dickinson et al. (1992a, b), and Dickinson and Metaxas (1994) used spatially global constraints, such as symmetry of an object (henceforth, spatially global constraints will be called "shape constraints"). These authors used them without making use of the formal-ism provided by regularization theory. Once they did not use regularization theory, they had to assume that shapes of real objects can be represented by a small number of simple components. This assumption was too restric-tive in the sense that it led to a working model that could only be used with objects that had simple components. Pizlo and his colleagues (Pizlo, Li, & Chan, 2005; Chan et al., 2006), working within regularization theory, were able to provide a model that could deal, at least in principle, with a greater variety of objects.

Pizlo and colleagues published results of a series of studies that tested the operation of several shape constraints in a shape constancy experi-ment. They used images of complex, unfamiliar polyhedral objects. These objects were designed in such a way that recognition of their shapes could not be based on identifying simple parts. Examples of stimuli used by Pizlo, Li, and Chan (2005) are shown in figure 4.9, and additional examples can be seen at http://viper.psych.purdue.edu/shapedemo. Each of these stimuli was produced from sixteen points, the vertices of a polyhedron. Only four of these were actually polyhedral objects (a, d, e, and f). Stimulus (b) shows only the sixteen points, and (c) shows these points connected in a random order to form a 3D polygonal line. The four types of polyhedral objects had different degrees of simplicity. Their simplicity (in decreasing order) was (a) a symmetrical polyhedron with planar contours, (d) a symmetrical polyhedron with some contours being nonplanar, (e) an asymmetrical polyhedron with planar contours, and (f) an asymmetrical polyhedron with nonplanar contours. Note that (d) and (e) are likely to have the same degree of simplicity because (d) is symmetrical but nonplanar, and (e) is asymmetrical but planar. Keep in mind that all six stimuli had a similar underlying 3D structure; they all are based on sixteen vertices of a poly-hedron. They differed only with respect to whether the points were con-

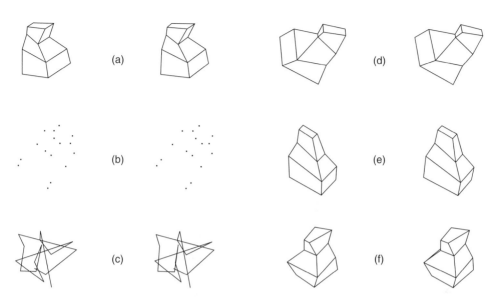

Figure 4.9
Stereoscopic images of stimuli in Pizlo, Li, and Chan's (2005) experiment.

nected, whether the object was mirror symmetrical, and whether its contours were planar. The stimuli in figure 4.9 were graded with respect to simplicity, stimulus (a) allowing the application of several shape constraints, but stimulus (c) allowing none. If shape constraints are necessary for shape constancy, performance in (a) should be the best and in (c) the worst. On each trial, the subject was shown two objects sequentially from different viewing directions, and the task was to decide whether the 3D shape of the two objects was identical. When the shape of the second object was different, the object was generated randomly. The subject was tested with all types of stimuli twice. Viewing was always binocular, but in one replication the images in the two eyes were identical, and in the other the images were disparate. As a result, binocular disparity could contribute to the three-dimensionality of the percept only in sessions where the images were disparate. There were a total of twelve sessions, one session per stimulus type and viewing condition.

Results of a naive subject are shown in figure 4.10. Results of the other two subjects, who knew the purpose of this experiment, were very similar. The graph shows the signal detection index of discriminability, d' (Macmillan & Creelman, 2005).[4] Higher values of d' represent better

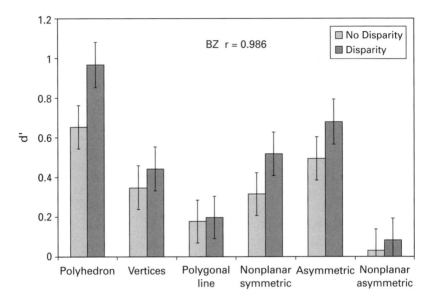

Figure 4.10
Results of one subject (B.Z.) in Pizlo, Li, and Chan's (2005) experiment.

performance. Performance was directly related to the availability of shape constraints: It was best for stimuli (a) and worst (close to chance) for stimuli (c) and (f). This was expected because when the object is structured, it allows for the application of constraints, and reconstruction can be performed. Otherwise, when the object is unstructured, reconstruction fails, as it did with the 3D polygonal line shown in (c), and with the nonplanar asymmetrical object in (f). Note also that when binocular disparity was available, performance was better than when it was not available. This difference was moderate, but statistically significant. What is important, however, is that perception of shape with binocular disparity is not reliable unless the perception of shape is reliable without binocular disparity (i.e., the same 2D stimulus is presented to both eyes). This can be clearly seen in (c), the polygonal line stimulus, as well as in (f), the nonplanar asymmetrical polyhedron. Once shape constraints could not produce a 3D shape percept from a single 2D image, binocular disparity contributed *nothing* to the perception of shape. These results strongly suggest that the perceptual mechanisms involved in the binocular perception of 3D shapes are very similar, if not identical, to those involved in the perception of 3D shapes from a single 2D image. In both, the 3D shape percept is produced by shape constraints.

The effect of shape constraints on shape constancy was tested in two additional studies with a wider range of stimuli (Chan et al., 2006), as well as with rotating 3D objects viewed monocularly (Pizlo & Stevenson, 1999). The results from these studies provided additional support for the role of shape constraints.

Pizlo, Li, and Chan (2005) and Chan et al. (2006) used the results of their experiments to develop a new model of 3D shape reconstruction. In this model, three shape constraints were used: planarity of contours, symmetry of the object, and minimum variance of angles (see section 4.4.1 for details of the model). Two of these constraints had been used before by Marill (1991) and Leclerc and Fischler (1992). Pizlo and his colleagues added the mirror symmetry constraint. Their model applies these three constraints to a single 2D retinal image to reconstruct a 3D shape. Once the 3D shape is reconstructed, the 2D image from the other camera (eye) can be used to correct the 3D shape. Chan et al. tested this model in simulation experiments with synthetic images, as well as with real images of a real 3D object (figure 4.11 shows an example). They also tested one of the standard models of shape from binocular disparity, in which shape constraints were not used. The accuracy of shape reconstruction produced by the new model was substantially higher than the accuracy of shape reconstruction based on binocular disparity alone. Furthermore, monocular performance of the new model was correlated with both monocular and binocular performance of the subjects in the shape constancy experiments.

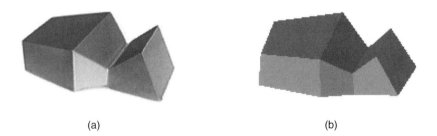

(a)   (b)

Figure 4.11
(a) An image of a 3D object. (b) An image of a reconstructed object (from Chan et al., 2006).

Binocular performance of the model, on the other hand, was not correlated with human performance. These results provide additional support for the claim that binocular and monocular mechanisms of shape perception are similar, if not identical. They both depend critically on shape constraints. The role of binocular disparity is secondary, at best.

To summarize, psychophysical research on shape perception during the last twenty-five years prepared the way for a new paradigm. It became clear that the percept of a 3D shape is not derived from the percept of depth. The information about depth, which is missing from the 2D retinal image, is made up by a priori constraints. A priori constraints are much more important in shape perception than in the perception of surface color, orientation, or motion because shape is much more complex as well as more structured than other perceptual attributes. In this, shape is unique.

5 A New Paradigm for Studying Shape Perception

The earlier chapters (i) organized a very large proportion of the existing knowledge about shape, (ii) called attention to and reconciled contradictions within this literature, and (iii) summarized psychophysical results, obtained with a wide variety of methodologies, more or less supporting a number of theories that varied widely with respect to their formalism. These chapters provided a number of conclusions about fundamental properties of shape perception that allow the introduction of a new paradigm for studying shape perception. This new paradigm begins by assuming that producing a 3D shape percept from a 2D perspective image(s) is computationally difficult and depends, critically, on the operation of a simplicity principle. Stated formally, shape perception should be treated as an ill-posed inverse problem whose solution requires using a priori constraints. In the new approach, the emphasis shifts from studying the role and interaction of depth cues to the nature and operation of constraints. Visual processing of shape begins with figure–ground organization. This establishes 2D shapes in the retinal image. Three-dimensional shapes are reconstructed from these 2D shapes.

5.1 Main Steps in Reconstructing 3D Shape from Its 2D Retinal Representation

Now that we know what has to be done, how can we do it? How can we reconstruct the 3D shapes from the 2D representation that we have on our retina? The first thing is to establish figure–ground organization within the 2D retinal image.

5.1.1   Establishing Figure–Ground Organization

Consider the 2D images in figures 1.2 and 1.3. These images illustrate the fact that figure–ground organization is as automatic and effective in line drawings as in photographs of the real objects used to produce the line drawings. These figures also show that objects are defined by the contours that give them shapes. Note that the objects are perceptually segregated from each other and from their background. Once figure–ground organization is established, it provides the observer with additional information. The third dimension is explicitly represented as soon as figure–ground organization takes place. The Gestalt psychologists pointed this out when they insisted that the contour belongs to the figure—it defines the object, which is perceived as being *in front of* the background. Note that once the object is perceived in front, it is being perceived as residing in a 3D space. However, with the impoverished stimuli the Gestalt psychologists used to make these points about figure–ground organization, the extent of the implied third dimension was marginal, at best. However, in real scenes, like those shown in figure 1.3, where there is more than one object present in the visual field, and where the objects themselves are structured, establishing figure–ground organization results in many more than two depth planes. We have known about the importance of figure–ground organization for about 100 years, since the Gestalt Revolution. Despite the fact that its importance has been known for a very long time, we are far from a full understanding of this phenomenon. We know that Gestalt grouping principles are important in shape perception, but there is no model that allows one to predict how 3D shape will be perceived in a variety of stimulating conditions. There have been a number of attempts in the machine vision community to do this, but there has been only limited success to date. The most promising approach will be described next.

Nevatia (2000) showed how this might be done. He took a photograph of a 3D scene, containing a number of common objects (figure 5.1a). His algorithm begins by finding pixels corresponding to gradients of intensity (this step is not shown in the figure). The next step is to group pixels into individual straight or curved line segments by using continuity and proximity constraints. This step is shown in (b). Note that this image is deceptive. The reader, looking at this image, can easily see the individual objects. This image looks a lot like figure 1.3. However, at this stage of the analysis,

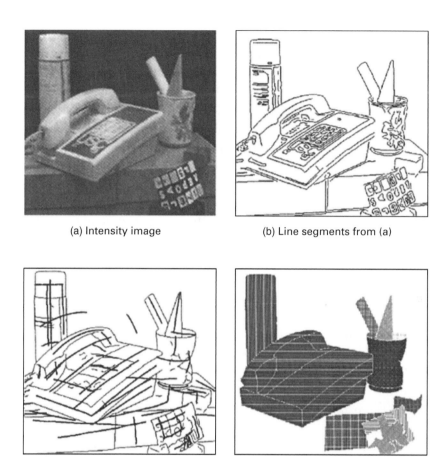

(a) Intensity image   (b) Line segments from (a)

(c) Selected axes of symmetry   (d) Segmented objects

Figure 5.1
Figure–ground organization using symmetry constraint (from Nevatia, 2000, figure 1.3, p. 180—with kind permission of the author and Springer Science and Business Media).

the algorithm does not know anything about the objects in the image. You do, but the algorithm does not. It only knows about individual lines that might represent the contours of objects. The third step, shown in (c), uses a symmetry constraint. It finds symmetrical groups of contours. They are represented by axes of symmetry marked by heavy lines. Symmetry, used in conjunction with a closure constraint, made it possible for Nevatia to represent individual objects, separated from the background and from each other. This is shown in (d). Clearly, the human visual system does a better job, but Nevatia's algorithm seems to be at least a promising first step in approximating what humans do so easily and accurately.

Why was symmetry so effective in establishing figure–ground organization? Symmetry is a common property of a wide variety of objects, ranging from bilaterally symmetrical bipeds like ourselves, and throughout the animal kingdom, to plants and trees, as well as to many inanimate objects (e.g., Thompson, 1942; Blum, 1973; Kanade & Kender, 1983).[1] All living creatures have been confronted by significant symmetrical objects throughout their evolution. If symmetry is both ubiquitous and informative, one should not be surprised to find symmetry providing a significant way to recognize or reconstruct objects "out there." Once so many different things "out there" tend to be symmetrical, many of their retinal images will be at least approximately symmetrical (Kanade & Kender, 1983; Jacobs, 2000). Furthermore, there is no good reason to expect that the contours of different, unrelated objects in the same visual field will form, by accident, very many approximately symmetrical configurations in the retinal image.

It must be emphasized, however, that figure–ground organization is far from being fully understood. There are, at present, no computational methods that can produce accurate figure–ground organization with real images of real scenes with anywhere near the accuracy of the human visual system. Nevatia's work does show that symmetry offers promise for establishing the figure–ground organization of the retinal image, but further elaborations are clearly necessary. Several suggestions for future research (human and machine) are listed below:

Human vision

(i) Study figure–ground organization in the context of 3D shape perception,

(ii) use realistic images of complex scenes, and

(iii) characterize the role of symmetry and mechanisms for detecting it.

Machine vision

(i) Use realistic images of complex scenes,

(ii) use images of unfamiliar objects, and

(iii) formulate models for efficient detection of symmetries in the 2D image.

Symmetry, once detected in the 2D image, is critical in reconstructing the 3D shape percept. However, any given 2D retinal image could be produced by very different 3D shapes. For this reason, the family of possible 3D percepts must be restricted before shape constraints such as symmetry are applied to produce the 3D shape percept.

5.1.2 Restricting the Family of Possible 3D Percepts

Once figure–ground organization has taken place, the question arises about how to transform the 2D image into a 3D percept. Constraints are needed. What is the nature of these constraints? One of the most important constraints—probably the most important constraint—for restricting the family of 3D percepts is called "planarity." Consider the example in figure 5.2. This polyhedral object was chosen because it is novel. It does not resemble anything you are likely to have seen before, so your percept of its shape could not have been affected by familiarity. Three perspective images are shown. All three are perceived as the same object despite its novelty. Note that this object is perceived as being composed of several faces located in different planes. The corners of the individual faces are perceived as coplanar. Coplanarity allows the visual system to perceive the object as having the same shape when viewed from different viewing directions (to demonstrate shape constancy). The importance of a planarity constraint for achieving shape constancy derives from the following two geometrical considerations. First, any perspective image of an object

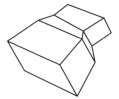 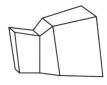

Figure 5.2
A polyhedral object seen from three different viewing directions.

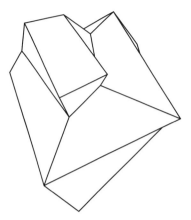

Figure 5.3
An image of a polyhedron whose contours are not planar.

consisting of planar faces permits a 3D reconstruction of an object with planar faces. Second, it is highly unlikely that a 3D object with faces that are clearly nonplanar will produce a perspective image that permits the reconstructed 3D object to have planar faces.[2] Figure 5.3 shows an image of an object whose contours are nonplanar. This image does not permit the reconstructed 3D object to have planar faces, and it is difficult to find an orientation of this object, relative to a camera, that would permit a planar interpretation.

Planarity is potentially important not only in the case of polyhedral objects, but also with objects that have smooth surfaces. Consider the examples in figure 5.4. This figure shows eight objects (generalized cones) whose shapes look very different (see chapter 4 for a brief discussion of generalized cones). Some of them are polyhedral, and others are not. Not only do these objects look different, but each can be recognized from most viewing directions. In other words, it is easy to achieve shape constancy with these kinds of shapes. Depth cues are not needed. The shapes of the objects can be veridically reconstructed from their symmetry. The use of symmetry in reconstructing 3D shapes will be discussed below. At this point it is important to realize that the planarity of some contours, as well as planarity of the axes of these generalized cones, substantially restricts the family of 3D shapes that are possible interpretations of a given 2D image. The reader will remember from the discussion of 2D perspective invariants presented in chapter 3 that the family of inverse perspective

Polygonal base   **Smoothly curved base**

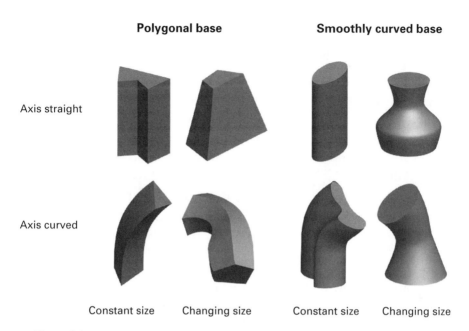

Axis straight

Axis curved

Constant size   Changing size   Constant size   Changing size

Figure 5.4
Examples of eight families of generalized cones (produced using 3DS Max/
Autodesk).

projections of a given 2D shape on the retina is characterized by only two
parameters, and the size of this family does not depend on whether the
shape is polygonal or smoothly curved. In the case of simple 3D polyhedra,
the family of inverse perspective projections is characterized by only three
parameters.[3] Clearly, if it can be assumed that some contours are planar in
the 3D shape, the family of possible 3D shapes will be small. Once the
family is small, it will be easy to apply shape constraints and reconstruct
the unique 3D shape percept. This will increase the likelihood of the shape
percept's being veridical.

The shape of each object in figure 5.4 can be described by a combination
of only a few characteristics: the shape of the base (cross section)—smoothly
curved versus a polygon; the shape of the axis—straight versus curved; and
the size of the cross section—constant versus changing. Note that these
characteristics can be determined based on a single 2D image of the 3D
object. This is why figure–ground organization is so important. It has to
be emphasized, however, that the examples in figure 5.4 are used only to
illustrate the main concept. The family of possible 3D shape interpretations

is not necessarily larger when the shape of the cross section is not constant and the angle between the cross section and the axis is not a right angle, as long as there are a sufficient number of planar contours. An example of such an object was shown in figure 5.2. This polyhedron is a generalized cone. It is substantially more complex than any of the cones in figure 5.4, but the family of inverse perspective projections produced by this image is characterized by only three parameters. The fact that only three parameters are needed results from the planarity constraint itself. Note that the object in figure 5.2 is symmetrical. More precisely, this object is bilaterally symmetrical. Interestingly, symmetry is a stronger 3D constraint than planarity. Namely, the family of symmetrical inverse perspective projections produced by this image is characterized by only one parameter (Vetter & Poggio, 2002; Li & Pizlo, 2007).[4] It follows that symmetry not only can be used to solve the figure–ground organization problem (see the previous section) and to establish a veridical shape percept (see the next section) but can also be used in the intermediate stage to restrict the family of possible 3D interpretations of a given 2D representation.

Note that the new paradigm for shape perception is quite different from the approach introduced by Biederman (1985). Biederman, using thirty-six "shape components," attempted to *recognize* shapes of real 3D objects. In the new paradigm, a 3D shape "out there" is *reconstructed* from its 2D retinal image. This reconstruction is accomplished by determining the family of inverse perspective projections of the object's 2D retinal shape, and by determining the 3D shape that minimizes a cost function, implementing a simplicity principle.

Now that the planarity constraint has been shown to be useful, one can ask whether it is ecologically valid. Said differently, could the planarity constraint be important in the perception of real objects in real environments, the goal set by Marr (1982)? It probably is for the following reasons:

(i) Many human-made objects are polyhedral, and for such objects, planarity of contours is trivially satisfied (e.g., tables, chairs, and buildings are fine examples of polyhedral objects with planar faces and coplanar corners).

(ii) Natural objects, such as animals and plants, are not like chairs. They do not have perfectly planar contours. However, at least some of their contours are approximately planar as indicated by Stevens (1981, 1986).

Stevens showed that if a surface can be approximated by a cylindrical surface (an assumption that is obviously true for human and animal limbs, as well as torsos), the lines of curvature are planar geodesics.

(iii) Any object with mirror symmetry has points and features that form planar configurations. This is because mirror symmetry of a quadruple of points implies the planarity of these points. Similarly, if a surface is locally symmetrical, then the symmetry line is locally planar (Weiss, 1988b).

(iv) Many 3D shapes, such as generalized cones, of the kind used by Biederman (1985) and Marr (1982), as well as Pentland's (1986) superquadrics, that were used in the past to model real objects, have symmetry axes, which themselves are planar curves or even straight lines.

(v) Developable surfaces that can be used to model surfaces of many objects can be characterized by straight lines that are geodesic lines.

In all these cases, a planarity constraint can be applied. It will considerably reduce the degrees of freedom in the family of inverse perspective projections.[5]

5.1.3   Achieving a Veridical Shape Percept

Now that we have seen that the planarity constraint is important in the perception of real objects in real environments, that is, it is ecologically valid, we can consider the third and final step in reconstructing a 3D shape from its 2D retinal image. Producing a 3D shape percept from a 2D retinal shape is accomplished by "adding volume" to the 2D shape. Note that adding volume to a 2D shape to produce a 3D shape percept must be constrained because there are, in principle, infinitely many possible 3D percepts of shapes for any given 2D retinal image, and only one of these possible percepts is veridical. We also already know that symmetry can play an important role in figure–ground organization and in restricting the family of possible 3D interpretations of a 2D image. It continues to be important when volume is added because *the 2D image will always be less symmetrical than the 3D shape that produced it*. The argument for the role of a symmetry constraint in shape constancy is analogous to the argument described for the role of planarity in shape constancy. Namely, *any* perspective image of a symmetrical object permits a 3D reconstruction of a symmetrical object. At the same time, it is highly unlikely that a 3D *asymmetrical* object will produce a perspective image that permits the 3D reconstructed object to be symmetrical. Thus, applying a symmetry constraint is likely

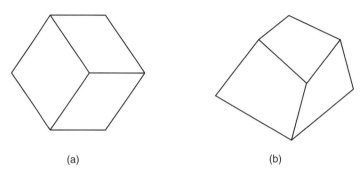

(a)   (b)

Figure 5.5
(a) An image of a cube. (b) An image of a box that is not exactly a cube (after Kanizsa, 1979).

to lead to a veridical percept. However, as the reader will see, symmetry, in itself, is not sufficient for the veridical perception of shape.

Consider the example shown in figure 5.5. Both (a) and (b) are perceived as 3D shapes, but only one of them is symmetrical—so, if the symmetry constraint is responsible for the percept in (a), what is responsible for the percept in (b)? It cannot be symmetry. It is probably limitations, such as this, of the symmetry constraint that encouraged Marill (1991) and Leclerc and Fischler (1992) to use alternatives to symmetry. They used a minimum-variance-of-angles constraint to reconstruct 3D polyhedral shapes (Marill used minimum variance of angles only, whereas Leclerc and Fischler used a planarity constraint, as well). Minimum variance of angles produced reconstructions that were somewhat similar to what a human observer perceives when shown a single image of a polyhedron. However, the minimum-variance-of-angles constraint is very limited. It can only be used with polyhedra. Most natural objects are not polyhedra. A more general constraint is needed. Before this can be done, another limitation of symmetry will be described because an effective constraint must deal with this additional limitation, as well.

Consider the examples in figure 5.6. The objects in (a) and (b) are perceived as rectangular boxes having identical 3D shapes. These 3D shapes have three planes of mirror symmetry. One might expect that it would be easy for a machine vision system to reconstruct these shapes by using a symmetry constraint. This is not the case with respect to (a) because (a) is not actually an image of a perfectly symmetrical rectangular box. It is an image of a box that is slightly asymmetrical. Note that the surface facing

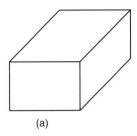   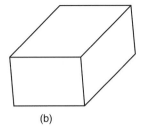

(a)   (b)

Figure 5.6
Both images are perceived as identical boxes, but only (b) is geometrically consistent with such an interpretation. Application of the symmetry constraint to (a) would produce an infinitely long rectangular rod. Reconstruction agrees with the percept when both the symmetry and compactness constraints are used.

the observer is a rectangle in the image. If it is a rectangle, the other two faces of the box would not both be visible from the observer's point of view. A human being confronted with this 2D image has no problem perceiving this box as a rectangular box. Using this 2D image, however, to reconstruct this 3D box cannot be accomplished by using a symmetry constraint. The 2D shape of the surface facing the observer is wrong. If a symmetry constraint is applied to (a), the result would be an infinitely long rectangular rod, whose long axis would be almost parallel to the line of sight. However, if the image of the surface facing the observer is not a perfect rectangle, as shown in (b), a rectangular box can be produced by applying a symmetry constraint. The bottom line here is that the symmetry constraint, when applied to two very similar retinal images, may reconstruct very different 3D shapes (reconstruction is computationally unstable). Thus, symmetry cannot be sufficient for solving the inverse problem of 3D shape reconstruction. One has to use at least one additional constraint to remove uncertainty in the 3D reconstruction (formally, to stabilize the solution of an ill-conditioned inverse problem). This problem can be solved by adding a compactness constraint. Note that a compactness constraint can be used with any object, not only with symmetrical or polyhedral objects.

The 3D *compactness* of an object is defined as V^2/S^3, where V is the volume and S is the total surface area.[6] Compactness of 3D shapes and of 2D shapes has been used in machine vision applications (see Bribiesca, 2000, and Ballard & Brown, 1982), but mainly as a tool for shape description, not for reconstruction.[7] When both compactness and symmetry are used in a cost function, and the cost function is applied to the images in figure 5.6, the reconstructed 3D shape is what the human observer perceives, namely, two similar rectangular boxes.

To summarize, in the new approach advocated here, 3D shape reconstruction relies on three main shape constraints: symmetry, planarity, and compactness. These three constraints become the essential element of a "new simplicity principle," according to which the perceived shape corresponds to the minimum of a cost function that represents the interaction between a 2D shape on the retina (produced by a 3D shape "out there") and a priori constraints applied to the 3D shape percept. Note that *this new simplicity principle is used because it leads to accurate 3D reconstructions, not because objects "out there" are simple.*

5.2 How the New Simplicity Principle Is Applied

The new simplicity principle permits reconstruction of a 3D shape from the available 2D image by using regularization theory. This is done by defining a cost function, whose minimum determines the perceived 3D shape. This cost function is the sum of two components, representing retinal information and shape constraints. It is analogous to the cost function that Poggio et al. (1985) used to reconstruct 3D surfaces. Recall that reconstructing surfaces involved applying spatially local constraints to the information provided by depth cues. In the new paradigm, reconstructing 3D shape involves applying spatially global (shape) constraints to the 3D retinal shape. The role of depth cues is secondary, at best. The first component of the cost function evaluates the degree of inconsistency between the reconstructed 3D shape and its 2D retinal image. For example, if the retinal image of a cube gave rise to the percept of a cube, consistency would be perfect. The consistency between the 3D percept and the 2D retinal image will never be perfect because there will always be some uncertainty associated with figure–ground organization. For example, in figure 5.6a, the reader perceives an elongated rectangular box. This percept is not consistent with the 2D image shown in this figure. The visual system can tolerate some inconsistencies between a percept and the available 2D retinal image. It tolerates this inconsistency in order to preserve the symmetry and compactness of the 3D shape percept. In the examples that will be given below, this term is ignored to simplify the presentation.

The second component of the cost function evaluates how well the a priori constraints are satisfied in the 3D shape percept constructed from the 2D image. In the new paradigm, this second component is responsible for making the 3D shape percept as symmetrical and as compact as possible.

Once both components of the cost function are specified, one is ready to use it to reconstruct 3D shapes. The reconstructed 3D shape is the shape that minimizes the cost function.

The rectangular box in figure 5.6b will be used to illustrate how a 3D shape can be reconstructed from its 2D image by using a symmetry constraint. The application of compactness will be illustrated later. Assume that figure–ground organization has already been performed, and the three closed contours representing the three visible faces have been identified in this 2D image. Furthermore, assume that a family of inverse perspective projections has been correctly determined by using the planarity constraint. In this case, the family is characterized by three parameters (see the discussion of figure C.11). Because only three faces are visible, the reconstruction of the 3D shape, obviously, can involve only these three faces. The reader should recognize that this aspect of the new reconstruction method resembles Marr's (1982) 2.5D sketch because his sketch represented only visible surfaces. However, this resemblance is superficial. There are two important differences between the new approach and Marr's approach. First, Marr reconstructs the visible surfaces from depth cues. The new approach does not use depth cues. Second, Marr represents the visible surfaces in the coordinate system of the viewer. The new approach represents the visible surfaces in the coordinate system of the object, the box in this case.

The next step in the reconstruction of the 3D shape from this 2D image is to apply a symmetry constraint. A rectangular box has several symmetries. The parallel faces have identical shapes, each face is a symmetrical 2D shape, and angles between all pairs of edges are right angles (90 deg). The departure of an object from symmetry in the polyhedral family, which contains this rectangular box, can be measured by how much the angles differ from right angles. In the 2D image shown in figure 5.6b, none of the angles are right angles. Six are acute, and six are obtuse. The same is true of every 3D object (except the rectangular box) in the polyhedral family, which can produce the 2D image shown in figure 5.6b. In all of these objects, some angles are acute and others obtuse. A rectangular box, however, is the only member of the polyhedral family where *all* angles are right angles. This means that this box represents the minimum of a cost function, measuring the departure from symmetry. It follows that identifying the minimum of the cost function will allow reconstruction of the 3D rectangular box from the 2D shape shown in figure 5.6b.[8]

Once the shape of the visible part of the box is reconstructed, the invisible, back part of the box can also be "reconstructed" by applying a symmetry constraint. It is sufficient to assume that the three invisible faces are symmetrical to the three visible faces. Interestingly, the invisible faces can also be reconstructed by using the planarity constraint. Sugihara (1986) pointed out that the 3D position of the invisible corner of a box is uniquely determined by the positions of the seven visible corners in figure 5.6b, once the planarity constraint is applied to the invisible faces. Clearly, the entire 3D shape of the object represented by the 2D image in figure 5.6b can be reconstructed without the need to use any 3D shape models stored in the memory, as Marr had claimed.[9]

Would the reconstructed shape be the same when the object is seen from different viewing directions? Would shape constancy be achieved? Figure 5.7 shows 2D images of the 3D rectangular box shown in figure 5.6b. When the cost function measuring departure from symmetry is applied to all of these 2D images, and when the 3D shape minimizing the cost function is identified, this 3D shape turns out to be the same for all of these different-looking 2D images. In other words, shape constancy would be achieved.

Symmetry and planarity constraints are sufficient in the case described just above in which figure–ground organization was assumed to be perfect. Once this assumption is not made, as would be required in the case of real

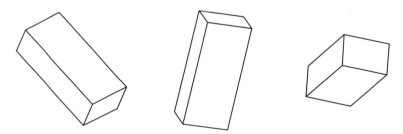

Figure 5.7
Three different views of the object from 5.6b.

images of real objects in real environments, an additional constraint is required for reconstruction. This issue was mentioned briefly in section 5.1.3 and illustrated in figure 5.6a. By way of reminder, symmetry and planarity can reconstruct polyhedra as long as symmetrical reconstructions are within the family of inverse perspective projections of a given 2D retinal shape. We also know that any uncertainty about figure–ground organization introduces errors that may preclude accurate reconstructions due to the instability of the reconstruction result. This problem can be overcome by introducing a compactness constraint. Compactness is defined as the volume squared, divided by the surface area, cubed (see above). When a cost function includes the compactness constraint, the boxes reconstructed from each of the two images in figure 5.6 are very similar to each other. This agrees with the percept. Shape constancy is achieved despite the less-than-perfect 2D retinal shape.[10]

Compactness and symmetry constraints also lead to accurate reconstructions with randomly generated symmetrical polyhedra, such as those shown in figures 4.4 and 5.2 (Pizlo, Li, & Steinman, 2006; Li & Pizlo, 2007). We generated several thousand synthetic wire objects. For each object, one 2D orthographic image was computed for a randomly chosen 3D orientation of the object. From each 2D image, we reconstructed a 3D object using symmetry and compactness constraints. Specifically, we computed a symmetrical object with maximal compactness. As pointed out by Vetter and Poggio (2002), a single 2D orthographic image of an object with one plane of symmetry is consistent with infinitely many 3D symmetrical objects (in other words, the problem is ill posed). This family of objects is characterized by one parameter, whose value cannot be determined from an image. The image does not contain enough information to produce a unique, let alone a veridical, reconstruction. The value of this parameter must be derived from a priori constraints. In our algorithm it is obtained by maximizing the compactness of the symmetrical object. The reconstructions were accurate or almost accurate for most objects and for most viewing orientations. When large errors occurred, the errors were quantitative, not qualitative. Specifically, the reconstructed object was wider or narrower than the original object, but the overall shape was very similar. Furthermore, it is worth noting that in the small number of cases in which the reconstruction was not accurate, the reconstruction tended to agree with the shape the observers perceived.[11]

This test was repeated with opaque objects. An opaque symmetrical polyhedron can be reconstructed when (i) at least three non-coplanar pairs of symmetrical vertices are visible and (ii) at least one vertex of the remaining symmetrical pairs is visible. Sixty percent of our randomly generated images of polyhedra satisfied these requirements (these images may be what Palmer et al., 1981, called "canonical views"). With 2D images satisfying the two requirements described just above, the entire 3D object can be reconstructed. The reconstruction is not confined to its front, visible part. The "back," hidden part of the object is reconstructed simply by applying symmetry and planarity constraints. It is important to note that the reconstructions of opaque objects were as accurate as the reconstruction of the transparent "wire" objects. Specifically, for more than 90% of cases, the error in the reconstructed depth was smaller than 20%, and the maximal error in the reconstructed depth did not exceed 50%. Once again, the errors that were observed were quantitative, not qualitative. All of these results have important implications for the role of depth cues in shape perception, in general, and for the role of cue combination, in particular, an issue discussed in detail in chapter 4. If the use of a simplicity principle suffices to explain shape constancy, depth cues may, and probably should, be left entirely out of the reconstruction because they are more likely to interfere with than contribute to the veridicality of the shape percept.

Next, the effectiveness of the application of this cost function will be illustrated with a well-known example from Shepard (1981). In the top portion of figure 5.8, 2D images of two different boxes are shown. These 2D images are perceived as having been produced by objects with different 3D shapes. What makes this example special is the fact that the *2D images* of the top faces of the boxes have identical shapes (one is oriented vertically in the image and the other horizontally). This is not a coincidence because the viewing orientations and the 3D shapes of the two different boxes were chosen in such a way that the top faces of their 2D images were identical. The reader, who surely will doubt this, should apply a ruler and a protractor to these 2D images or, even better, trace one of the two top faces and superimpose it on the other. Clearly, these two parallelograms are not perceived as having identical shapes, despite the fact that the shapes of their 2D images are identical. This example shows that we cannot see our retinal images, a point frequently made by the Gestalt psychologists. These 2D images represent two different 3D objects (i.e., there is no

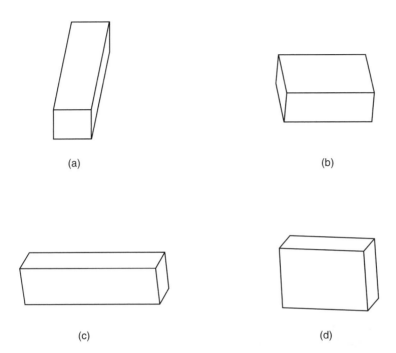

Figure 5.8
(a) and (b) are perceived as different 3D objects. In particular, the top faces are perceived as different 2D shapes, even though these two parallelograms are identical on the 2D image (from Shepard, 1981—with kind permission of Lawrence Erlbaum Associates). (c) and (d) are different views of the 3D objects shown in (a) and (b) when the objects were reconstructed using symmetry and compactness constraints.

object that could produce these 2D images when viewed from different viewing directions), and we see these objects as different (the 3D shape percept is veridical, not illusory). When the new approach is used to reconstruct the 3D objects from these 2D images, the cost function predicts what you actually see (the cost function was the same as in the previous example—see note 10). Different views of these two 3D objects are shown in figure 5.8c and 5.8d. Here, there is no surprise because from these viewing directions, the faces in front are no longer the same shapes in their 2D images. Once this is appreciated, two things stand out. First, one should not be surprised. Second, the new simplicity principle works very well.

Next, consider how well the new simplicity principle works with real objects whose shapes are more complex than the boxes Shepard used.

Compactness is easy to compute for boxes. But how about more complex objects such as the human body, or objects that do not have volume? Look at the 3D object, a chair, shown in figure 5.9a. This object has little volume. In such cases one may compute compactness for a box circumscribed on the chair (figure 5.9d). Note that it should be possible to specify the 2D image of this box because the chair and its parts are symmetrical. In other words, the box defines a natural, object-centered frame of reference for the chair (Marr, 1982; Palmer, 1985, 1999). Once this box is defined, one can apply the cost function to the box rather than to the chair. Figures 5.9b and 5.9c show two views of the chair reconstructed from the image in (a) when the cost function was computed in this way. Clearly, the reconstruction agrees quite well with the percept produced by looking at (a), and it agrees with the 3D shape of the chair that was used to produce (a). A similar

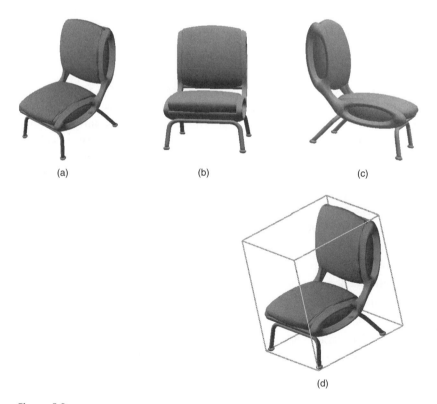

(a)   (b)   (c)

(d)

Figure 5.9
(a) An image of a chair. (b) and (c) Two views of the reconstructed chair. (d) A rectangular box used in the 3D reconstruction (from turbosquid.com).

result was obtained for a 3D object depicting a man. The image used for reconstruction is shown in figure 5.10a, and two views of the reconstructed object are shown in (b) and (c).

It has to be pointed out that these two examples involving complex objects were used to illustrate only one step in the 3D shape reconstruction. Namely, they illustrated that the minimum of a cost function involving two shape constraints applied to a circumscribed 3D box corresponds to the perceived 3D shape of the inscribed complex object. This step, applying shape constraints, was discussed in section 5.1.3. The other two steps, figure–ground organization and determining the restricted family of inverse perspective projections (sections 5.1.1–5.1.2) were not applied to these examples. As a result, in these two examples, the cost function was actually applied to different 3D transformations of the 3D chair and the 3D man rather than to their 2D images (the family consisted of 3D affine transformations of the circumscribed box and of the complex objects that are consistent with the given 2D image). Obviously, the first two steps, establishing figure–ground organization and determining the restricted family of possible 3D shape percepts, are not trivial. Future research must address not only these three steps individually but also the

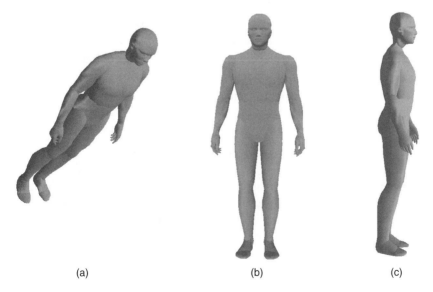

(a)   (b)   (c)

Figure 5.10
(a) An image of a man. (b) and (c) Two views of the reconstructed man (from turbosquid.com).

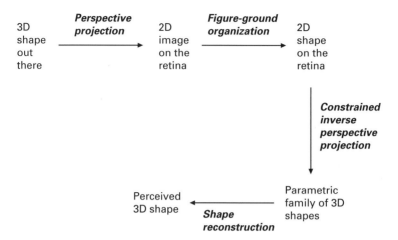

Figure 5.11
The steps involved in shape constancy.

quality of the shape constancy achieved by the complete reconstruction model (see figure 5.11).

A final note: Many complex objects, such as animals and humans, consist of parts, such as torsos, arms, and legs, and the individual parts can move independently (the entire object is only piecewise rigid). A number of attempts to deal with complex objects like these have been made in the past with limited success. The best known was that of Biederman (1987), who dealt explicitly with shapes of parts of objects, not with the shapes of entire objects. He recognized the potential importance of the Gestalt-like simplicity principle but applied it locally rather than globally. In his words,

Recognition-By-Components posits a specific role for these organizational phenomena in pattern recognition . . . the Gestalt principles, particularly those promoting Prägnanz (Good Figure), serve to determine the individual geons, rather than the complete object. A complete object, such as a chair, can be highly complex and asymmetrical, but the components will be simple volumes. . . . If the components can be recovered and object perception is based on the components, then the object will be recognizable. (1987, p. 126)

Simplicity was used in his approach only by limiting the number of simple components. He used a symmetry constraint only at the level of the parts, not at the level of the object. However, natural objects are more often than not symmetrical, and they have a natural frame of reference determined by such features as symmetry, elongation, and gravity (Rock, 1973; Marr, 1982; Palmer, 1985, 1999). These aspects of complex shapes may allow the reconstruction of 3D shapes independent of the shapes of the parts. A giraffe is likely to look like a giraffe, even if it has horse's legs. Once the 3D shape is reconstructed, its parts and their 3D relations can be specified quantitatively by using methods like those presented by Pelillo, Siddiqi, and Zucker (1999), Siddiqi et al. (1999), Sebastian, Klein, and Kimia (2004), and Ioffe and Forsyth (2001). This means that one should be able to recognize a 3D shape regardless of the particular orientation of its parts, relative to one another. For example, in the case of a human body, when posture changes, the 3D shape of the body and the shapes of its parts can be reconstructed independent of one another. This allows recognition that it is still a human body. In other words, shape constancy would be achieved.

To summarize, a great deal is known about human shape perception. However, we are far from having a complete understanding of the perceptual mechanisms involved. That this is true follows trivially from the fact that there is no machine vision system whose performance comes close to the performance of human observers. It is possible to assemble a machine vision system that produces unreliable performance and demonstrates illusions that mimic illusions like those produced by the human visual system, but much more work is needed to find out how the human visual system achieves shape constancy, not how it fails. This effort is most likely to require collaborations between the human and machine vision communities.

It was unclear how much more work would be needed to formulate a "complete theory" of shape perception when the first draft of this book was completed. Progress made within the last several months has made it obvious that the approach described in this book was proceeding in the right direction. The idea of "inflating" the 2D shape to produce a 3D shape by using the new simplicity principle worked very much better than had been anticipated (see the previous section). The success of the new simplicity principle in reconstructing 3D shape from a 2D image meant that the new theory of shape perception, which is summarized in the next section, is much closer to a "complete" theory than could have been anticipated only a few months ago. The new theory will be summarized by contrasting it with the main prior attempts to "explain" shape perception.

5.3   Summary of the New Theory

The new theory provides a plausible explanation of how shape constancy is achieved in human vision. This new theory of shape constancy is also a theory of shape perception *because* shape constancy is the sine qua non of shape. To put it in everyday language, there is nothing about shape perception that cannot be demonstrated in a shape constancy experiment. This claim, which runs contrary to common wisdom, has been developed, explained, and justified throughout this book. Its main argument can be summarized as follows. Shape has nothing to do with the viewpoint of an observer because the shape of an object is intrinsic to the object. It follows that the only way to be sure that one is studying shape, rather than depth or the orientation of surfaces, is to study shape constancy. Depth and the orientation of surfaces depend on viewpoint. Shape does not.

Depth and the 3D orientation of surfaces were emphasized in Marr's theory, a theory that provided the most widely accepted explanation of shape constancy since its introduction in 1976. In Marr's theory, 3D shape was derived from the 3D orientations of surfaces. Using conventional terminology, shape constancy was achieved by "taking context into account," the same explanation that has been used to explain all other constancies, but in all constancies other than shape, context was critical because the retinal image was always *ambiguous*. Shape is different from all other perceptual properties because shape is *complex*. It is easy to see that shape's complexity prevents shape ambiguity. Namely, shapes of different objects are very unlikely to produce identical retinal images. In other words, s*hape ambiguity is very rare*, so shape constancy, unlike size, depth, position, lightness, color, or speed constancy, can be achieved *without making any use of context*. This makes shape *unique*. The new theory of shape perception presented in this book is built on this important fact.

Complexity, with its resulting uniqueness, has not played a role in any prior theory of shape perception. Marr did not use it, nor did Gibson. Biederman recognized that shape is unique, but he emphasized the *simplicity* of shapes, not their *complexity*. The 3D percept of shape in Biederman's theory depends critically on the shapes of his "geons'" being simple. Complexity, in Biederman's theory, only plays a role at a later stage when objects are recognized.

Another way to contrast Marr's theory with the theory described for the first time in this book is to look at the relation between surfaces and volume in both theories. In Marr's theory, surfaces are computed first. Volume comes in later. In the new theory described here, volume is established first, and the surfaces around it result from computations of the shape's "maximal volume." In the new theory, unlike in Marr's and in almost all other shape theories, the three-dimensionality of the percept is not derived from depth cues. Instead, the three-dimensionality of the shape perceived is *assumed* by the visual system. This assumption, which is based on a priori knowledge of the environment, seems to be intuitively obvious. It can be thought of as an instantiation of the Law of Prägnanz introduced by the Gestalt psychologists. *Why should the visual system waste computational resources in order to determine that a 2D retinal image was produced by a solid object when all 2D images in the evolutionary history of our species have been produced by solid 3D objects!*

Most objects important to humans allow a great deal of shape constancy to be achieved. There are exceptions, however, where we know that constancy is likely to fail, even when the object is complex. These failures raise two questions, namely, what are these objects like and what is the significance of the failure to achieve shape constancy when they are present in the environment? Shape constancy is likely to fail with unstructured objects such as a ragged rock, a crumpled newspaper, a potato, or a casually folded piece of fabric. It is certain that an observer can perceive the surfaces of such objects despite the fact that he or she cannot perceive their shapes. We know that the shapes of such unstructured objects cannot be perceived *because* shape constancy fails when they are used in constancy experiments (see chapter 4). Recall that when constancy fails, it fails because no unambiguous shape is available to the observer. Why should there be any ambiguity left after shape constraints are applied to the 2D images of such 3D objects? Ambiguity remains because in the case of unstructured 3D objects like these, shape constraints may be ineffective. They may be ineffective simply because there will be infinitely many possible solutions when one tries to find the most symmetrical and most compact 3D shape possible with the 2D images that objects like these produce on the retina (see chapter 4). In such cases, the surfaces of a 3D object are perceived, but its shape is not. Note that in the new theory, unlike in Marr's, surfaces are not closely tied to shape. Surfaces *are* perceived by taking depth cues into account, whereas shapes are perceived as a result of the operation of "shape priors." It should not be surprising that when shape constancy fails, objects are perceived and recognized by using information about their surfaces. Is the absence of shape likely to cause problems in identifying such unstructured objects? The answer is probably "no" because there is no unique shape that can characterize any unstructured object like those described above. Some of these objects (fabric or newspaper) are nonrigid, and their shapes can change arbitrarily. In the case of others, shape is not informative at all because there is no 3D shape shared by all potatoes or by all rocks. Clearly, shape constancy seems to fail only with objects whose shapes cannot be used to identify them or to discriminate one from another.

Is this new theory of shape likely to lead to a complete explanation of shape constancy? There is considerable reason for optimism. The simulation experiment on the reconstruction of random polyhedral shapes, reported by Pizlo et al. (2006) and Li and Pizlo (2007) and described in the previous section, strongly suggests that symmetry and compactness constraints are sufficient for veridical reconstructions of the shapes of structured objects. The strength of this experiment lies in the fact that it used randomly chosen unfamiliar objects. Using unfamiliar objects is critical for testing shape constancy in both humans and machines because if you use a familiar object, such as your car, one can argue that you see its shape veridically because you have seen it many times from many viewing directions. A weakness of the Pizlo et al. experiment, however, is that the randomly chosen stimuli are "unnatural." This raises a significant question, namely, how likely is it that the results of a shape constancy experiment with such "unnatural" objects will generalize to the shapes of natural objects, such as the bodies of animals or fruits? There are two good reasons for optimism.

First, if our "unnatural" stimuli were processed by different visual mechanisms than processed natural stimuli, it seems unlikely that the "unnatural" stimuli used in the Pizlo et al. experiment would have demonstrated near perfect shape constancy. Nearly perfect shape constancy can be demonstrated with natural objects in everyday life as well, as in the laboratory. Parsimony alone seems a sufficient reason to accept the assumption that the visual mechanisms used to process both "unnatural" and natural stimuli are at least very similar, perhaps even identical. Second, natural objects such as the bodies of animals and fruits are nearly symmetrical. Furthermore, they tend to be "maximally compact." It was shown (above) that symmetry alone can drastically reduce the family of possible 3D interpretations of a 2D image to, at most, a few degrees of freedom. This is completely analogous to how the "unnatural" randomly chosen polyhedra, used by Pizlo et al., were reconstructed by application of the new theory. It is true that application of symmetry constraints is relatively easy when distinctive points are provided, as they were with the polyhedral objects used in the Pizlo et al. experiment. However, symmetry constraints can also be applied to natural objects having fewer distinctive points. Unfortunately, at present, computational geometry is not sufficiently developed to allow us to do these computations efficiently, if at all. But this deficiency is not the first, nor the last, example of the fact that there is more to visual (perceptual) geometry than can be found in existing textbooks on machine vision.

Now that we have seen that (i) the three-dimensionality of the percept does not have to be derived from retinal images, but can simply be assumed, and (ii) a veridical 3D shape percept can be produced simply by the application of symmetry and compactness constraints, it becomes clear that the most difficult aspect of 3D shape reconstruction has been explained. It follows from these considerations that it should be possible to make machine vision systems that perform as well as, perhaps even better than, humans perform in shape perception tasks. Recall that figure–ground organization establishes the contours and regions in the 2D retinal image that represent individual 3D objects "out there" (see section 5.1.1). In the new theory of shape constancy, figure–ground organization is followed by an intermediate stage during which the parametric family of 3D inverse perspective projections is established (see section 5.1.2). Working out the details of these two stages is difficult, but work is under way and progress is being made as this is being written. Now that the goal of these two stages can be stated clearly, namely, providing appropriate input for the shape priors to operate, formulating a plausible model may be relatively easy. Keep in mind that up to now the important role that figure–ground organization *must* play in shape perception was not appreciated. Now that its role can be stated clearly and now that we have developed a very effective simplicity principle, it should be possible to move rapidly toward our goal

of understanding how human beings perceive naturalistic shapes veridically in realistic environments. It even should be possible to make a
machine that can do this too.

The best way to appreciate where we are is to summarize how we got
here. This will be done by summarizing what it took to achieve our current
understanding of shape perception by tracing the obstacles that had to be
overcome (millstones) and the signposts signifying success **(milestones)**
on the road to understanding shape.

5.4   Millstones and **Milestones** Encountered on the Road to Understanding Shape

5.4.1   The "Taking Slant into Account" Explanation of Shape Constancy during the Heyday of Empiricism (1083–1912)

The first explanation of shape constancy was assumed to be the same as
the explanation of other constancies, namely, constancy was explained by
taking into account the context in which the critical feature of the stimulus
appeared. For example, in the perception of 2D shapes, the slant of the
shape's surface provided the context. This explanation was especially
favored by the empiricists, which means that it was accepted by most
people interested in shape perception before 1912 when the Gestalt Revolution began. The "taking slant into account" explanation was one of the
main millstones impeding progress toward developing an understanding
of shape constancy. Note that understanding shape constancy is essential
for understanding shape itself.

At the end of the nineteenth century, Helmholtz proposed an alternative
explanation that did not make use of slant. For Helmholtz, the perception
of shape was based on memorizing a large number of 2D views of a given
object. The mechanism described by Helmholtz made use of an "unconscious conclusion." The observer "inferred" the shape of the object from
its retinal image and the memory of previously seen images of the same
or similar objects. This nineteenth-century theory resembles a contemporary look-up table type of explanation, in which associations between
retinal stimuli and 3D percepts are established by learning. Although it did
not receive much attention when it was first presented, Helmholtz' look-up
table theory was often used (usually without attribution to him) in the
1990s as a model for machine vision (Poggio & Edelman, 1990), as well as

for a theory of human shape perception (e.g., Edelman & Bülthoff, 1992).

5.4.2 Thouless' (1931a,b) Experiments, Ostensibly on Shape Constancy, Actually Studied Shape Ambiguity

Unfortunately, this first attempt to study shape constancy in psychophysical experiments used ellipses as stimuli. This family of shapes is characterized by only one parameter (its aspect ratio). Ellipses are not sufficiently complex to be used as stimuli to study shape (the family of triangles is also unsuitable). Perspective projection changes 2D shapes with two degrees of freedom, which means that Thouless actually studied shape *ambiguity*, not shape *constancy*. His results pertain to depth, not to shape, perception. Thouless did establish that depth cues improve the perception of a slanted ellipse. This result, which was subsequently replicated with triangles, does not generalize to *any* other 2D shape. Thouless has been, repeatedly and mistakenly, credited for establishing that shape is perceived by "taking slant into account." Had Thouless been correct, the "taking into account" principle could have been used to "explain" all perceptual constancies. He was wrong, however. Shape is special because it is complex and requires its own theory. The shape ambiguity/shape constancy confound introduced by Thouless (1931a,b) resurfaced twice in the 1990s—first, when shape constancy was studied with unstructured stimuli such as polygonal lines (e.g., Rock & DiVita, 1987), and then again in binocular experiments on the perception of the depth of simple 3D objects (e.g., Johnston, 1991).

5.4.3 The Gestalt Psychologists Make Progress by Introducing a Simplicity Principle and Figure–Ground Organization (1912–1935)

The first breakthrough in studying shape came with the Gestalt psychologists, who emphasized that the percept cannot be explained by analyzing the content of the retinal image. They claimed that the perception of shape requires the operation of a simplicity principle. According to this principle, the shape most likely to be perceived is the simplest possible interpretation of the retinal shape produced by a 3D object "out there." It would take more than half a century and many arguments and controversies involving individuals working in the Gestalt and Empiristic traditions before this view was accepted and a computationally useful version of this critical principle was formulated.

A 3D shape percept cannot be produced until its 2D shape on the retina is established. Establishing 2D retinal shapes is called "figure–ground organization." Calling attention to the importance of figure–ground organization is the second critical contribution of the Gestalt psychologists. Figure–ground organization and the underlying simplicity principle have been studied extensively, but the role of this principle in 3D shape perception was greatly underestimated until recently. Additional work on figure–ground organization is needed before we can make effective use of this critical initial stage in models of human and machine visual systems. The human visual system organizes the 2D retinal image into figures (the 2D shapes of objects) and backgrounds much faster and much better than any machine system devised to date. In fact, there is currently no machine vision system that can do it at all when realistic images are used. Understanding the former should make appreciable improvements of the latter possible.

5.4.4 Stavrianos (1945) Publishes an Experiment that Actually Demonstrates Shape Constancy

Stavrianos used rectangles to study shape constancy. This is the simplest family of shapes that avoids shape ambiguity because *four* parameters are required to characterize the shape of a rectangle. Ellipses and triangles are not sufficiently complex for shape constancy to be achieved because they have too few parameters. Stavrianos showed that shape constancy can be obtained and that achieving it does *not* involve making use of cues to depth. This was the first legitimate experiment on shape constancy, but its significance went unnoticed for a very long time. The shape constancy achieved without depth cues in Stavrianos' experiment can be explained by the use of perspective invariants.

5.4.5 Studying Shape Thresholds and Shape Illusions Adds Little (1920–1970)

A simplicity principle can be used to make up for information lost in the perspective projection from a 3D scene to the 2D retina. This fact means that the role of a simplicity principle that can do this is best studied with 3D shapes. A simplicity principle is *not* needed for the perception of a 2D shape. A simplicity principle *is* needed to establish figure–ground organization, the process that produces 2D shapes on the retina, but, when the shape percept is 2D, no information is missing. Gestalt psychologists, and those they influenced, tried to demonstrate the operation of a simplicity principle by (i) studying the conflict between the simplicity principle and the retinal image and (ii) studying interactions between shapes and the contexts that produced a new class of illusions called "figural aftereffects" (Köhler & Wallach, 1944). Clearly, a simplicity principle is needed to understand shape perception. However, it is important to keep in mind that this simplicity principle is used by the visual system to *add* information lost during the transformation from 3D to 2D, not to compete with the 2D image. Thus, devoting effort to studying 2D shape thresholds and shape illusions was a blind alley. It added little, if anything, to our understanding of either shape perception or shape constancy.

5.4.6 Cognitive Psychologists (1953–1976) Make Progress by Shifting from the Study of 2D Shapes to the Study of 3D Shapes and by Shifting Their Interest from Simplicity to Veridicality

Formulation of information theory was one of the main factors leading to the Cognitive Revolution. Information could now be measured, and the complexity of messages could be quantified. If one conceptualizes shape as a message, its simplicity could be measured. The interest in information theory stimulated new research on shape despite the fact that the analogy between shapes and messages is far-fetched. Fortunately, interest at this time shifted from 2D to 3D shapes. When the main function of shape becomes allowing the identification of an object, 3D shapes become interesting; 2D shapes are not interesting in the real world because real objects are always 3D. From this point on, research on shape perception focused on 3D shapes. By the end of this period, it was widely recognized that the visual system uses a simplicity principle to produce veridical percepts. Percepts are of no use to the observer if they are not veridical. Recognizing this represented appreciable progress toward developing an understanding of shape constancy, as well as of shape itself.

5.4.7 Progress Is Inhibited When Empiricism Is Revisited (1947–1983)

The Cognitive Revolution was stimulated by increased interest in neuroscience as well as by the introduction of information theory. The progress in electronic instrumentation achieved during World War II, had an immediate effect on neuroscience, leading to systematic study of the architecture of the visual system. The conceptual background for this work was provided by Hebb in his influential book published in 1949. He provided a neo-empiristic theory of visual perception in which all visual percepts, even those as elementary as the percept of a line segment, were learned. The learning mechanism proposed by Hebb was borrowed from Pavlov's conditioning theory. For a number of reasons, neural neo-empiricism contributed little, if anything, to our understanding of shape.

Other neo-empiricists in this period concentrated on the role of cognitive factors in perception, with a special emphasis on learning and thinking. They took the Gestalt simplicity principle and reformulated it as a likelihood principle. The main figure in the neo-empiristic camp, Rock, gradually drifted away from the likelihood principle toward the traditional empiristic position represented by the "taking into account" explanation of shape constancy. The main difference between Rock and his empiristic predecessors was that Rock assumed that shape constancy involves thinking, not just stimulus–response relations. Neglecting both simplicity and likelihood principles, and emphasizing learning and thinking, was a "giant step" backwards.

5.4.8 Progress Is Made by Using Computational Models in Machine Vision (1965–1982)

By around 1970, the study of human vision had reached an impasse. There were several very different and conflicting theoretical approaches, called "direct perception," "unconscious inference," "neo-Gestalt," and "perceptual learning." It was not clear how one was to choose among them. An answer came from the machine vision community. All in the human vision community at that time assumed that producing a 3D shape percept is fairly easy, but how this was done differed among the various approaches. It was commonly accepted in this period that explaining veridical perception was easier than explaining illusions (e.g., Braunstein, 1976, p. 174), so many in the vision community concentrated on studying illusions. This concentration on illusions was only put to rest when the machine vision community tried to simulate the operation of veridical perceptual mechanisms on a computer. By the early 1970s it had become clear that explaining veridical perception is actually extremely difficult, far harder than simulating human illusions. It is so difficult that without the "existence proof" provided by the success of the biological vision systems, the machine vision community would surely have agreed that the goal of creating a general purpose vision system, which perceived veridically, was well beyond reach.

5.4.9 The Unfortunate Neglect of Figure–Ground Organization (1950–1985)

Two influential contributors, Gibson and Marr, claimed that there was no need to include the perceptual organizing principle the Gestalt psychologists called "figure–ground organization" in their theories of 3D shape and space perception. Their reasons were quite different. Gibson claimed that a priori rules of perceptual organization are not needed because veridical visual perception is simple (Gibson, 1950, p. 196). Marr ruled out figure–ground organization because it was too difficult to implement in a computational model. The consensus achieved by these two influential, but clearly not like-minded, scientists, kept the study of figure–ground organization separate from the study of 3D shape perception.

5.4.10 Gibson's Putative "Direct" Perception (1950–1979)

Gibson, despite being impressed with the importance of veridicality and ecological validity in visual perception, adopted a Fechnerian position in which the percept requires only sensory coding. No additional higher level processing is needed. Thus, according to Gibson, a simplicity principle is not needed, learning is not needed, and computations are not needed. We just see things as they really are. Gibson's commitment to naive realism had a lasting effect in the human vision community despite the fact that it must have been obvious by the late 1970s that this approach could not explain shape perception, nor many other perceptual accomplishments. Gibson did appreciate the fact that veridical perception is important and illusory perception is not. However, his failure to appreciate the fact that the veridical perception of shape is a computational problem routinely solved by the visual system kept him, from contributing anything of merit to shape perception. The next step was taken by others. Gibson's idea, called "direct perception," is equivalent to treating perception as a forward (direct) problem. The fact that perception is an inverse problem was only explained by Poggio et al. (1985) after Gibson died. This shift in emphasis opened the way for progress.

5.4.11 Marr's Paradigm: The "Taking Slant into Account" Principle Revisited (1982– . . .)

Marr offered a 2.5D sketch as a substitute for figure–ground organization. Shape was important for Marr, but surfaces were even more important. Marr wore his mathematical hat when he formulated his theory. Once one realizes that the "curvature," a derivative of the orientation of a surface, can be used to describe the surface's shape, it seems to follow naturally that the visual system should derive shape from orientation. Marr did not appreciate how difficult it would be to reconstruct surfaces. At the same time, he failed to recognize the uniqueness of shape. Marr's approach was almost surely motivated by Julesz's introduction of random-dot stereograms with which 3D shapes could be perceived without providing any shapes in the stimuli. Julesz made an important contribution when he showed that binocular disparity itself, in the absence of any other cues, can produce the percept of depth relations. However, there is a long way to go from generating shapes with random-dot stereograms to understanding or reconstructing the shapes of natural objects from their 2D images. Note that random-dot stereograms are not common in our natural environment, so there is no reason to expect that the primary mechanism of 3D shape perception is the one that begins with computing binocular disparities rather than 2D shapes on the retina. Breaking visual camouflage, a visual ability similar to fusing random-dot stereograms, may be important, even critical, for predatory animals or for the military reading aerial photographs, but not for ordinary human observers in everyday life. If disparity were to be essential for perceiving shape in everyday life, any of our ancestors who lost an eye would have been at a great disadvantage. Humans now, and most likely then, manage very well with a single eye. There seems to be little reason to afford binocularity, disparity, and random-dot stereograms a critical role in natural shape perception.

5.4.12 Marr's Neglect of Psychophysical Experimentation

Marr strongly influenced the vision and cognitive science communities when he introduced his three-level approach to the analysis of a biological system. The first level in his approach is the development of a computational theory, which specifies *what* is to be computed and *why* it should be computed. His second level specifies *how* these computations are to be performed. This is called the "algorithmic" level. His third level describes neuroanatomical and neurophysiological implementations of the algorithm. The second level can be tested in psychophysical experiments. The third level can be tested in neuroanatomical and neurophysiological experiments. But how did Marr propose to test his first "computational" level? Marr never explicitly stated whether or how a computational theory should or could be tested experimentally. Perhaps he was planning to test it after the other two levels had been examined in some detail, or perhaps he believed that his computational theory of shape in which surfaces are reconstructed (the *what* part) in order to see objects (the *why* part) is self-evident. It seems rather unusual that empirical verification of an important claim like this was not high on Marr's list, a fact that is not without consequences for the scope and power of Marr's theory of shape perception. All of the efforts of Marr and his group were devoted to formulating algorithms of what they called "shape from X" (where X represented a depth cue such as disparity, motion, shading, or texture). These algorithms should have been called "surface from X" rather than "shape from X." Some effort did go into psychophysical tests of individual algorithms (e.g., algorithms for binocular stereopsis), but no effort went into testing the computational theory itself. Marr probably simply ran out of time because of his untimely death. The absence of such tests held back, one could even say misdirected, the study of shape for thirty years.

5.4.13   Important Steps, but in the Wrong Direction: Projective Invariants and a Model Based on an Uncalibrated Camera (1988–1995)

Once the idea of "invariants" appeared in the vision literature (thanks to Gibson, who used the term frequently but inconsistently and often incorrectly), the machine vision community explored what and how much can be done with "invariants." *Projective* invariants were the only invariants that could be applied to perspective images that were known in mathematics at the time. Using projective invariants is based on the assumption that the human eye is an uncalibrated camera. This assumption is not correct. The human eye is a calibrated camera: Its focal length and the position of the fovea are "known" to the human visual system. As a result, projective invariants cannot be used to model human vision. Specifically, shapes that "look" identical to projective invariants may look very different to a human observer. Using the terminology of signal detectability, projective invariants produce higher false-alarm rates in a shape recognition task. Put differently, projective invariants would make shape ambiguity an important problem, perhaps even as important as shape constancy. The reader should realize by now that this would be undesirable, to say the least. Progress clearly required appreciating the fundamental limitations of projective invariants. An appreciation of these limitations led to the development of a new kind of invariants, called "perspective invariants," and to the acceptance of the "calibrated camera" as the appropriate model of the human eye.

5.4.14 Progress Produced by Introducing Perspective Invariants and a Calibrated Camera Model (1990–...)

A calibrated camera is the appropriate model for the human eye. In particular, the visual system "knows" both its focal length and the position of the fovea. Such a camera is able to use all the information present on the retina. This model is mathematically less convenient than the model provided by an uncalibrated camera, but it is unquestionably the appropriate model to use to study human vision. The properties of a calibrated camera model had actually been in practical use for a long time, but their implications for projective geometry had never been made explicit. Once they were made explicit, it became clear that conventional mathematical invariants (projective and affine) do not provide a complete description of the geometry of perspective projection in the human eye (Pizlo & Rosenfeld, 1990, 1992; Pizlo, Rosenfeld, & Weiss, 1997a, b). The formulation of new invariants, called "perspective invariants," was very important. It (i) provided a long-overdue explanation of Stavrianos' (1945) results on shape constancy with 2D figures, (ii) paved the way for the formulation of model-based invariants, (iii) called attention to the importance of the complexity of shape and the lack of relevance of depth cues, and (iv) set the stage for formulating a plausible model of shape constancy with 3D shapes.

5.4.15 The New Paradigm of Inverse Problems (1985–...)

Introducing the paradigm of inverse problems and regularization theory was a turning point in the history of perception. This paradigm changed the way perception, in general, and shape perception, in particular, has been studied and modeled. In this paradigm, perception is a difficult inverse problem that cannot be solved without a priori constraints. A priori constraints are at least as important as traditional visual cues. This new paradigm revived Gestalt ideas one more time. Recall that it was the Gestalt psychologists who emphasized that the retinal image is not sufficient to explain the percept and who first introduced the concept of a priori simplicity constraints. The translation of these vague ideas into formal computational models was triggered by the introduction of the paradigm of inverse problems to vision science (Poggio et al., 1985). Currently, all serious efforts in mathematical and computational modeling of vision involve regularization or Bayesian models. When the new paradigm was introduced, it was considered to be an extension of Marr's paradigm. This, by itself, was a millstone, but, considering all of the implications that followed from its introduction, the inverse problem paradigm deserves to be classified as one of the most important milestones, leading to the development of an understanding of shape perception.

5.4.16   The Role of Depth Cues in Shape Perception: The "Taking Slant into Account" Principle Emerges One More Time (1987–...)

The popularity of Marr's 2.5D sketch was responsible for the way most human vision has been studied for many years. Marr assumed that the depth and orientation of surfaces were the key to understanding shape perception. However, depth and orientation judgments are very unreliable. This made it plausible to assume that shape perception would be unreliable, too. This proved to be the case, but only (i) when impoverished, unstructured stimuli are used and/or (ii) when the viewing orientation of the object relative to the observer is severely restricted. Each of these choices has fatal consequences for the study of shape. The use of unstructured stimuli was motivated by attempts to study the relation between shape and depth uncontaminated by regularities of objects, such as their symmetry. But leaving out all of the regularities that natural objects have naturally resulted in leaving shape completely out of the stimuli used in putative studies of shape! The second choice, restricting the viewing orientation, was motivated by attempts to study, as directly as possible, the relation between Marr's 2.5D sketch (the 3D percept in a viewer-centered representation) and the shape (the 3D percept in an object-centered representation). But, if only one viewing orientation is used, shape constancy cannot be studied, and shape constancy is the best (perhaps the only) basis upon which one can be sure that one is studying shape rather than some other property of the test stimuli. Also, if only one viewing orientation is used, one learns little about how shapes of objects are recognized in everyday life. In everyday life, objects are seen from different viewing directions because the human observer often changes his or her position relative to the environment, to say nothing of the fact that many significant objects in natural environments change their orientation with respect to the human observer.

5.4.17   Memorizing 2D Images of Objects in Order to Recognize 3D Shapes: Empiricism Revisited (1990– . . .)

The fact that the percept of a 3D shape is itself 3D has not been questioned for a long time. However, the difficulty inherent in developing a computational model that could recognize at least some shapes from real images encouraged some researchers to ignore 3D perceptual representation altogether and to study the perception of 3D shape by providing extensive training with 2D images of 3D objects. The idea that 3D shapes could be recognized by memorizing a series of 2D representations originated with Helmholtz (1867/2000). The machine vision community gave it new credibility in the 1990s, more than 100 years after it had been proposed by Helmholtz. This multiple-views theory is analogous to Gibson's, despite many differences between the two. Both are wrong for a similar reason. Gibson assumed that the 3D world maps *directly* to the 3D percept. Proponents of the multiple-views theory assume that the 2D retina maps *directly* to the 2D percept. Gibson left out the retina, while the 2D multiple-views theorists left out the third dimension from the percept. Both theories treated perception as a direct (forward) problem rather than as the inverse problem it is now known to be.

5.4.18   The Importance of Figure–Ground Organization Is Finally Recognized (1985– . . .)

Those few individuals who did not confine themselves to Marr's 2.5D sketch after its introduction in 1976 explored the role of figure–ground organization. Progress was extremely slow because this problem is very difficult. Establishing 2D shapes in a noisy image of a cluttered naturalistic environment is challenging. There has been continuous progress in understanding this problem and appreciating its difficulty within the machine vision community since the middle of the 1980s. Progress started with models of 3D shape recognition, in which the establishment of a fast and efficient percept of the shapes of 3D objects was assumed to be based on perceptual grouping's leading to contours and shapes in the image (Biederman, 1985; Lowe, 1985). This early computational work showed, once again, that this problem was very difficult and that "smarter" methods for establishing 2D shapes were needed. Today, very few would dare to doubt that figure–ground organization plays a critical role as the first step to establishing a 3D shape percept. Specifically, figure–ground organization is critical because it establishes 2D shape on the retina and prepares the way for 3D shape reconstruction by means of shape constraints. Once it is recognized that Marr's 2.5D sketch was adopted to substitute for understanding figure–ground organization, it should be easier to remove the 2.5D sketch from theories of shape now that figure–ground organization is back in the picture.

5.4.19 The Uniqueness of Shape Is Finally Recognized (1985–...)

The fact that shape is unique was recognized by the human vision community only twenty years ago. Once the uniqueness of shape had been recognized, the human vision community began to (i) study shape constancy with complex stimuli whose shape had more than one or two parameters and (ii) determine the experimental conditions required for shape constancy to be achieved reliably. It became clear very quickly that 3D shapes can be, and are, perceived veridically. They can be perceived as one and the same shape from many viewing directions. Attempts to treat shape as a unique perceptual property were few and far between, and they were immediately faced with fierce opposition. There were two main reasons motivating this opposition. First, many human vision researchers insisted on confusing shape constancy with shape ambiguity. The former requires shape to be special; the latter does not. Second, all attempts to formulate a working computational model that used a 3D representation of shape failed, whereas some limited success was achieved by models that used a 2D shape representation. Progress in machine vision is evaluated by comparing one's own algorithm to the algorithms of one's predecessors; it is not based on whether any of the algorithms actually work (see appendix C, section C.1a). Despite these failures, appreciation of the fact that shape constancy is of fundamental importance and that shape is special, taken in conjunction with progress in understanding figure–ground organization and the acceptance of inverse problems theory, paved the way for a new paradigm. There was only one element missing, namely, the concept of shape constraints.

5.4.20   Recent Misguided Attempts to Change the Conventional, Meaningful Definition of Shape Constancy (1990– . . .)

The most recent conceptual millstone was an attempt to change the conventional, unambiguous definition of shape constancy to a definition that leads to experiments that have nothing to do with shape. Conventionally, "shape constancy" refers to the fact that the percept of the shape of a given object remains constant despite changes in the shape of the object's retinal image. Said slightly differently, the retinal image changes when the orientation of the object relative to the observer changes, but the perceived shape of the object does not change; it remains constant. Suppose you conduct an experiment in which neither the retinal shape nor the percept of the shape changes. Does this kind of experiment have anything to do with what is conventionally called "shape constancy"? How about an experiment in which the retinal shape does not change but the perceived shape does? Can this experiment be interpreted as a failure of shape constancy? A number of contemporary researchers have answered "yes" to both questions (e.g., Doorschot et al., 2001; Nefs et al., 2005; Scarfe & Hibbard, 2006). Doing this, of course, completely changes the conventional meaning of shape constancy. Accepting this change would be going back to the confusion that led to Thouless' misleading experiment published in 1931. Shape constancy cannot present itself when the retinal shape does not change, regardless of whether or not the perceived shape changes. If the retinal shape is not changed in the experiment, shape ambiguity, not shape constancy, is being studied. Thouless (1934) claimed that shape constancy is not a reliable perceptual phenomenon and even proposed that it should not be studied when he failed to observe constancy in an experiment that used stimuli with an insufficient number of parameters to allow constancy to manifest itself. Recently, a number of investigators, including those cited above, have proposed treating shape constancy and shape ambiguity as one and the same phenomenon. This is not a good idea either. We will be much better off concentrating on explaining shape constancy rather than denying its existence. We should also avoid confounding shape constancy with shape ambiguity. Shape constancy and shape ambiguity are different phenomena in several ways, namely,

(i) shape constancy, unlike shape ambiguity, is common in everyday life; (ii) retinal shape, figure–ground organization, and a priori shape constraints are critical in shape constancy, but not in shape ambiguity; and (iii) cues to depth and to orientations of surfaces, context, and familiarity are critical in shape ambiguity, but not in shape constancy.

5.4.21 The Role of Shape Constraints in Reconstructing 3D Shapes (1991–. . .)

The concept of shape constraints had been emerging slowly. By shape constraints we mean an a priori simplicity principle involving spatially global aspects of 3D objects, such as symmetry or compactness. The concept of shape constraints appeared for the first time with Gestalt psychologists, who did not use this term (Kopfermann, 1930). It was elaborated by neo-Gestalt psychologists in the 1950s, 1960s and 1970s. It was then used by the computer graphics community to provide informal models of the human 3D shape percept (Marill, 1991; Leclerc & Fischler, 1992). Shape constraints were also used in models of shape recognition (Biederman, 1985; Pentland, 1986; Dickinson et al., 1992a). The role of shape constraints in shape constancy could not be fully appreciated, however, before the importance of figure–ground organization was recognized. This required rejecting Marr's 2.5D sketch. Also, shape constraints could not lead to plausible models of shape constancy before the introduction of the formalism of inverse problems. However, note that this formalism had to be applied to shape, not to surfaces as Marr and his followers had done. All of these considerations only became clear a decade ago (Pizlo & Stevenson, 1999; Pizlo, 2001). Since they became clear, a growing number of psychophysical and simulation experiments have provided strong support for the new paradigm, in which shape constraints have played a critical role in the reconstruction of 3D shape.

In conclusion, progress toward understanding shape was made whenever it was recognized that the perceptual property called "shape" was unique. The main concepts that led to this progress, figure–ground organization and the simplicity principle, were formulated long ago by the Gestalt psychologists. It took more than seventy years before these ideas were implemented by the machine vision community in the form of computational models. Clearly, the contributions of the machine vision community were critical, but only when this community became aware of, and took seriously, what had been worked out and what was known in the human vision community. All attempts to understand shape outside of the context provided by psychophysical results on shape constancy led investigators astray. Keeping this in mind as our research proceeds should, in time, allow us (i) to understand how the human visual system achieves shape constancy with real objects in natural scenes and (ii) to make a machine visual system that works as well as our own.

Considerable progress has been made in developing this new theory of shape perception since the manuscript was sent to the publisher in the Spring of 2007. Specifically, a computational model has been developed that can recover the 3D shape of a symmetrical polyhedron from one of its 2D images. An additional shape constraint has been incorporated into this model. This new constraint minimizes the total surface area of the recovered shape. It has never been used before in 3D shape recovery. Using a weighted combination of the maximum compactness and minimum surface constraints recovers 3D shapes more accurately than using either alone. Furthermore, these recovered shapes are very similar to the shapes perceived by human observers presented with the same 2D stimuli. We also now know that the shape recovered by the model is quite stable in the presence of image noise and that the recovery can be performed from most viewing directions. The family of shapes that can be recovered includes all polyhedral objects with mirror symmetry, as well as many other symmetrical objects in which characteristic points can be identified. Demonstrations illustrating the success of this elaborated new model are available on the author's website (http://viper.psych.purdue.edu/~pizlo/). A detailed formal treatment of the model is also available there.

Appendix A: 2D Perspective and Projective Transformation

A.1 Perspective Projection Representing Retinal Image Formation of 2D Figures

This section is based on the material published in Pizlo and Rosenfeld (1992). A perspective projection between two planes is defined by six parameters. The position and orientation of one of these planes (the image plane) can be fixed without loss of generality. Let the equation of this plane be $Z = f$. This means that the image plane is orthogonal to the Z-axis and its distance from the origin of the XYZ coordinate system is f. This plane will be called the "image plane." The position and orientation of the second plane (called the "object plane") relative to the image plane is specified by three parameters. Its 3D orientation is represented by slant and tilt. Slant (σ) is the angle between vectors normal to these two planes, and it is in the range between 0 and 90 deg. Since the Z-axis is the normal to the image plane, it follows that slant is the angle between the Z-axis and the normal to the object plane. Tilt (τ) is the angle between an orthographic projection on the XY plane of the normal to the object plane and the X-axis. Tilt is in the range between 0 and 360 deg. Use of slant and tilt is not the only way to characterize the orientation of the object plane, but it seems that the visual system uses this parameterization (Stevens, 1983). It is worth pointing out that this parameterization is somewhat counter-intuitive. The reader should not be discouraged when he or she first tries to understand it. Understanding perspective projection is essential for understanding shape perception, so making a special effort to understand this parameterization is worthwhile. Figure A.1 illustrates this parameterization. One way to understand the meaning of tilt and slant is to realize that tilt specifies the orientation of the axis of rotation of the object plane relative to the image plane (tilt is orthogonal to this axis) and slant

τ = 0 deg   τ = 45 deg   τ = 90 deg

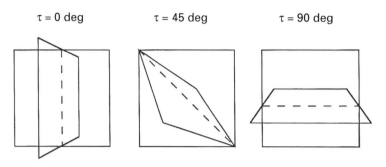

Figure A.1
Tilt is the direction of slant (from Pizlo, 1994).

specifies how much the object plane is rotated away from the image plane. The position of the object plane is specified by the distance C of the intersection of the object plane with the Z-axis from the origin of the coordinate system. Finally, the 3D position of the center of projection V is specified by three parameters, namely its 3D coordinates. Here, V is assumed to coincide with the origin of the coordinate system. A perspective mapping between the two planes (image and object) is established by the lines going through the center of the projection.

In the human eye, the nodal point is the center of the perspective projection and the retina corresponds to the image plane. Obviously, the retina is not planar (flat). However, from the point of view of the information obtained by the visual system, the shape of the retina is not important, as long as the visual system "knows" the shape of the retinal surface. The reasoning underlying this claim goes as follows. Assume that the image plane is tangent to the retina at the center of the fovea. It is obvious that the visual rays, that is, the lines going through the nodal point in the eye, establish a one-to-one mapping between the retina and the image plane. This means that even though the actual images on the spherical retina are different from the corresponding images on the image plane, they provide the same amount of information because one can always compute one image from another, as long as the shape of the retinal surface is known. From now on, we will assume that the retina is represented by the image plane. In the human eye and in any camera, the center of projection is located between the object and its image. Since the Z-axis is usually assumed to point toward the object, it follows that f is negative. It is not uncommon, however, to use a positive f in computations. Physically, this does not make sense because a camera with the image plane in front of the lens would not produce any image. Mathematically, however, the only effect of changing the sign of f is that the retinal image is right side up, rather than upside down. This corresponds to changing the sign of both x and y coordinates in the image. This is just one of many examples where mathematical convenience does not have any physical interpretation. In this particular case, this does not cause any problems, but in some other cases, using mathematical convenience has caused problems in attempts to study shape (see chapter 3).

Next, we need to specify the coordinate systems on the image plane and on the object plane. Let the x-axis on the image plane be parallel to the X-axis, and similarly, let the y-axis on the image plane be parallel to the Y-axis. Finally, let the point $(0,0,f)$ be the center of this coordinate system. The choice of the coordinate system $x'y'$ on the object plane is a little tricky. Pizlo and Rosenfeld (1992) used a coordinate system for the object plane, which led to simple formulas, but whose graphical interpretation was not simple. Here we will do the converse. Let the point $(0,0,C)$ be the center of the coordinate system on the object plane. As a result, the origin of the coordinate system on the object plane is projected to the origin on the image plane. We define the coordinate system on the object plane when slant is zero (in such a case, tilt is undefined). Let x' be parallel to x and y' parallel to y. The object plane with its coordinate system $x'y'$ for an arbitrary slant and tilt is produced by rotating this plane around the line that goes through the origin and is orthogonal to the tilt direction by an angle equal to slant. The perspective projection from the object plane to the image plane is specified by the following formulas:

$$x^* = x' \cos \tau + y' \sin \tau,$$
$$y^* = -x' \sin \tau + y' \cos \tau. \tag{A.1}$$

$$x = f \frac{x^* \cos \sigma \cos \tau - y^* \sin \tau}{x^* \sin \sigma + C},$$
$$y = f \frac{x^* \cos \sigma \sin \tau + y^* \cos \tau}{x^* \sin \sigma + C}. \tag{A.2}$$

It can be seen that the distance f between the center of projection and the image plane is a multiplicative factor in perspective projection. By changing it, the size but not the shape on the image plane changes. The distance C between the object plane and the center of projection, however, has a nonlinear effect on the image. Increasing C changes both size and shape on the image plane. This means that for a given figure on the object plane, its retinal shape changes with $3df$: σ, τ, and C. However, if the retinal size is fixed, the retinal shape can change with only $2df$: σ and τ. It can also be seen that if the size of figure on the object plane is changed by the same factor as the viewing distance C, the image remains the same. This will be clear when we write equations for inverse perspective projection.

It can be shown that the set of perspective projections is not a group (see chapter 3 for a definition of a group of transformations). Specifically, a composition of two perspective projections (i.e., a perspective projection followed by another perspective projection) is not, in the general case, a perspective projection. Instead, it is a projective transformation. This can be verified by applying equations (A.1–A.2) twice and verifying that the resulting equations have more terms in the numerators and in the denominator. These equations take the form described in section A.2.

Equations (A.1) and (A.2) can be used as a computer graphics tool because they allow one to compute perspective images of planar figures. For example, if one wants to run a psychophysical experiment on perception of planar figures that are slanted in 3D, then the images can be computed using equations (A.1) and (A.2) and displayed on a computer monitor. The computer monitor should be orthogonal to the subject's line of sight. The distance between the subject's eye and the computer monitor should be represented in equation (A.2) by f, and f should be positive. Note that f must be expressed in the same units as the image on the computer monitor. This means that the computer monitor must be calibrated by measuring how many pixels correspond to 1 cm. Then, one takes the figure whose image is to be computed and decides about slant, tilt, and distance C. For simplicity, C may be equal to f. Again, the figure itself and the distance C must be expressed in the same units as f and the image on the computer monitor. Figure A.2 shows two examples. Figure A.2b is a perspective image of (a) with slant 60 deg and tilt 30 deg when the viewing distance was fairly large. Figure A.2c is a perspective image of (a) with slant 55 deg and tilt 180 deg when the viewing distance was fairly small. Despite (or perhaps because of) the simplicity of equations (A.1) and (A.2), they are not readily available in textbooks.

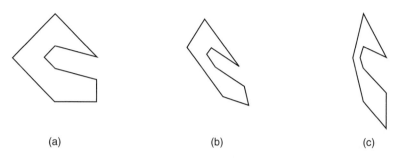

(a)   (b)   (c)

Figure A.2

(b) is a perspective image of (a) with slant 60 and tilt 30 deg for a large viewing distance ($E = 2$ deg). (c) is a perspective image of (a) with slant 70 and tilt 180 deg for a small viewing distance ($E = 30$ deg).

Note that a "perspective projection" between two planes, which refers to a one-to-one mapping between points of the planes, can be specified without coordinate systems on the planes. However, in order to write down equations representing the relations between the object and the image planes, coordinate systems have to be chosen.

It is instructive to write equations for an inverse perspective projection, that is, for a projection from the image plane to the object plane. This can be done by expressing $x'y'$ as a function of xy:

$$x^* = C \frac{(x\cos\tau + y\sin\tau)/\cos\sigma}{f - x\tan\sigma\cos\tau - y\tan\sigma\sin\tau},$$

$$y^* = C \frac{-x\sin\tau + y\cos\tau}{f - x\tan\sigma\cos\tau - y\tan\sigma\sin\tau}.$$

(A.3)

$$x' = x^*\cos\tau - y^*\sin\tau,$$

$$y' = x^*\sin\tau + y^*\cos\tau.$$

(A.4)

Equations (A.3) and (A.4) are useful when the task of the interpretation of the retinal image is considered. In a sense, one can say that the human visual system uses these equations. Note that the viewing distance C does not affect the shape of the figure "out there." Because the distance f is fixed in the human eye, it is clear that shape perception involves only two degrees of freedom: slant and tilt. Equation (A.3) is particularly important because it will be used in chapter 3 to derive invariants of perspective projection.

A.2   Projective Transformation of a Plane

2D projective transformation between xy and $x'y'$ planes is specified by the following equations:

$$x' = \frac{ax + by + c}{gx + hy + i},$$
$$y' = \frac{dx + ey + f}{gx + hy + i}. \tag{A.5}$$

Note that the denominators in the two equations are identical. There are a total of nine parameters, but only eight are independent. At least one of the following three must not be equal to zero: g, h, or i. We can then divide the numerators and denominators by this parameter, without changing the ratio.

Since a 2D projective transformation has $8df$, the projective transformation is uniquely defined by a transformation of four points, no three of which are collinear. And conversely, any quadruple of points can be projectively transformed to any other quadruple of points (no three of which are collinear). This means that all stimuli (rectangles) in Stavrianos' experiment, as well as their perspective images (trapezoids), were projectively equivalent. In other words, in 2D projective space, there is only one quadrilateral.

It is easy to show that the mapping (A.5) represents a group of transformations. Note that equation (A.2) has the form of equation (A.5) except that some terms are missing. It follows that a 2D projective transformation is more general than a 2D perspective projection. In both, perspective projection and projective transformation, straight lines are mapped to straight lines.

A.3   2D Projective Invariants

It is known that every group of transformations has its corresponding invariants. In the case of 2D projectivity, the invariant is represented by a pair of cross ratios. Take five points, A, B, C, D, and E, no three of which are collinear (the invariant cannot be computed when only four points are given, which means that projective invariants cannot be applied to Stavrianos' stimuli). We can compute areas of triangles represented by any triplet of points. We then compute a ratio of ratios of areas as follows:

$$I_1 = \frac{S_{ABD}S_{BCE}}{S_{BCD}S_{ABE}},$$

$$I_2 = \frac{S_{ABD}S_{ACE}}{S_{ACD}S_{ABE}}.$$

(A.6)

The cross ratios in equation (A.6) are derived from determinants of points, which means that the areas of triangles can be either positive or negative depending on whether the points *ijk* form a clockwise or a counterclockwise cycle. After any 2D projective transformation of a plane, as defined by (A.5), the pair of values (I_1, I_2) remains unchanged for any five points, no three of which are collinear. And conversely, if a 2D transformation of five points leaves the values (I_1, I_2) unchanged, it means that these five points are projectively equivalent (Rothwell, 1995). This means that the pair of values (A.6) allows a unique recognition of figures under 2D projective transformations. Consider a simple example. Take a set of N projectively different pentagons that were seen in the past. They can be "remembered" by storing for each of them a pair of values (A.6). Then, a projective (or a perspective) image of one of the pentagons is presented. Assuming that the correspondence of the five vertices is known, we can compute (I_1, I_2) for this image (a projective transformation of a pentagon is a pentagon). This pair of values will uniquely determine which (if any) of the N pentagons stored in the memory is presented. This means that the invariant (A.6) can be used to recognize projectively different pentagons (or more generally, n-gons, $n > 4$). If Stavrianos used pentagons, rather than quadrilaterals, in her shape constancy experiment, her results might have been consistent with projective invariants. By using quadrilaterals (rectangles), she "rejected" a theory based on projective invariants. Stavrianos was not aware of this.

Appendix B: Perkins' Laws

B.1 Derivation of Perkins' Law

Take the angle γ in figure 2.4. This angle is an image of an angle γ_0, which is assumed here to be equal to 90 deg. Let $\vec{L_2}(x_{L_2}, y_{L_2}, z_{L_2})$ and $\vec{L_3}(x_{L_3}, y_{L_3}, z_{L_3})$ be legs of γ_0. Let the z-axis coincide with the visual axis. Let $\vec{l_2}(x_{L_2}, y_{L_2})$ and $\vec{l_3}(x_{L_3}, y_{L_3})$ be the orthographic projections of $\vec{L_2}$ and $\vec{L_3}$ on the image plane (x and y coordinates of L are equal to the corresponding coordinates of its orthographic projection l). The following relations hold:

$$\vec{L_2} \cdot \vec{L_3} = L_2 L_3 \cos(90°) = 0 = x_{L_2} x_{L_3} + y_{L_2} y_{L_3} + z_{L_2} z_{L_3}, \tag{B.1}$$

$$\vec{l_2} \cdot \vec{l_3} = l_2 l_3 \cos \gamma = x_{L_2} x_{L_3} + y_{L_2} y_{L_3}. \tag{B.2}$$

From the two relations, we obtain:

$$l_2 l_3 \cos \gamma + z_{L_2} z_{L_3} = 0. \tag{B.3}$$

And, from this we obtain:

$$-\cos \gamma = \frac{z_{L_2} z_{L_3}}{l_2 l_3}. \tag{B.4}$$

Equation (B.4) is equivalent to equation (1) in Perkins and Cooper (1980). Without restricting generality, we can assume that $0 \leq \gamma \leq 180$. It follows that the left-hand side of equation (B.4) is negative when γ is acute and positive when γ is obtuse. The denominator on the right-hand side of equation (B.4) is always nonnegative (it is zero only in degenerate cases). The numerator on the right-hand side is positive (γ is obtuse) when z_{L_2} and z_{L_3} have the same sign. This happens when both $\vec{L_2}$ and $\vec{L_3}$ point away from or both point toward the observer. With three edges emanating from a common vertex of a right trihedral angle, either all three have the same direction (away from or toward the observer) or two of them have the same direction. It follows that in the image of a right trihedral angle, either all three angles are obtuse or one is obtuse and two are acute. The line drawing in figure 2.4 satisfies this criterion, whereas that in figure 2.5b does not.

B.2   Perkins' Rule under Perspective Projection

In a perspective image of a parallelepiped, at least one set of four edges, which are parallel in 3D space, are not parallel in the image. However, the lines containing images of all these edges must intersect at a single point, called a "vanishing point," if the box is a parallelepiped. In the case of figure B.1a, images of each of the three sets of four edges intersect at a

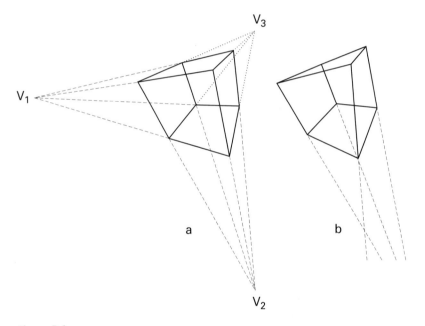

Figure B.1
(a) A perspective picture of a cube. When the reader keeps this figure at a distance equal to the size of the picture, the retinal image is also a perspective picture of a cube. Images of edges that are parallel in 3D are on straight lines that intersect at a single (vanishing) point (V_1, V_2, and V_3). The percept corresponds (approximately) to a cube when the face containing the left-most corner is perceived in front. The other, depth-reversed interpretation is very different from a cube. (b) A perspective picture of a box that is not a cube, not even a parallelepiped. This can be verified by drawing straight lines through the images of the four "vertical" edges of the box. These four lines do not intersect at a single point.

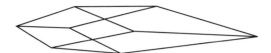

Figure B.2
A perspective image of a cube that does not look like a cube. The cube was in the far periphery of the camera that took this picture (after Pizlo & Scheessele, 1998).

point, but this is not true with one set in figure B.1b. This means that these four edges are not parallel in 3D space, and thus, the object that produced this figure is not a parallelepiped. It is not, therefore, a rectangular parallelepiped, either.

However, adding this criterion for determining whether a perspective image was produced by a parallelepiped is still not strong enough. It is not strong enough because this rule applies to any perspective image, that is, any image obtained by an eye with an arbitrary focal distance and an arbitrary position of the principal point (fovea). *However,* in the human eye, the focal distance and the position of the fovea are *not* free parameters; they are constant. This means that some perspective images of 3D scenes *cannot* be obtained on an actual human retina (Pizlo, 1994; Pizlo et al., 1997a, b; Pizlo & Scheessele, 1998). This is illustrated in figure B.2 which is a perspective picture of a cube but does not look like a cube. When the observer fixates at the center of the picture shown in figure B.2 and when the picture is orthogonal to the line of sight, the retinal image within the eye is identical to this picture except for its size. The point, here, is that this retinal image is not a valid projection of a cube, even though it is a perspective image of a cube. This retinal image could have been produced by a cube if the human eyeball had a different focal distance, that is, it had a different diameter, and if the fovea was not near the center of the retina. The fact that this figure does not look like a cube suggests that the human visual system "knows" the intrinsic geometrical parameters of its eye, such as its focal distance and foveal position. A combination of knowledge of the geometry of the eyeball and knowledge of the rules of perspective projection is sufficient for rejecting a parallelepiped interpretation when this interpretation is not consistent with the retinal image. Pizlo and Loubier (2000) formulated a criterion for deciding whether a given retinal image is a valid projection of a given 3D object. Their criterion can be applied to any 3D object, not only to a parallelepiped.

Appendix C: Projective Geometry in Computational Models

C.1a   Methodological Differences between Human and Machine Vision

Human Vision	Machine Vision
The goal is to learn how the mind works.	The goal is to build machines.
Progress in the field is evaluated by comparing the ingenuity of researchers to the ingenuity of nature.	Progress in the field is evaluated by comparing the ingenuity of researchers to the ingenuity of other researchers.
Researchers study a system that works, but they do not understand how (yet).	Researchers understand the systems they have built, but the systems do not work (yet).
A theory of the system is formulated after making thousands of observations of the system's performance.	A theory of the system must be formulated before even a single observation of the system's performance can be made.
The field provides lots of results but few theories.	The field provides lots of theories but few results.
Researchers often concentrate on one detail of the system.	Researchers usually work on large parts of the entire system.

This table is included to make it easy for the reader to understand why machine vision has not played a larger role in research on human vision to date. However, more importantly, understanding the limitations implied by these differences should make it easier for researchers in both fields to understand each other.

C.1b   Types of Geometrical Invariants Relevant to Shape Constancy

Projective invariants   properties (a ratio of ratios of distances or of surface areas) that are not changed by a perspective projection or any sequence of perspective projections of a 2D shape (Klein, 1939).

Affine invariants   properties (a ratio of distances of parallel line segments or of areas) that are not changed by a parallel projection. Affine invariants can also be used in the case of a perspective projection or any sequence of perspective projections of a 2D shape as long as the angular size of the projected shape is small.

Perspective invariants   properties (ratios of distances in a ψ function representation) that are not changed by a perspective projection of a given 2D shape onto the image in the eye or in a calibrated camera (Pizlo & Rosenfeld, 1992).

Model-based projective invariants   properties (a ratio of ratios of distances or of volumes) that are not changed by a perspective projection or any sequence of perspective projections of a limited class of 3D objects, namely, polyhedra or cylinders of revolution (Rothwell, 1995).

C.2   Perspective Projection from 3D Space to a 2D Image

Consider the XYZ coordinate system, whose origin coincides with the center of projection of the camera (nodal point of the eye). Let the image plane of the camera (surface of the retina) coincide with the plane $Z = f$ and the origin of the camera coordinate system xy (center of the fovea) coincide with the point $(0,0,f)$.[1] Finally, let the axes x and y be parallel to the axes X and Y, correspondingly. A perspective (retinal) image of an object point $V(X,Y,Z)$ can be computed as follows:

$$x = f\frac{X}{Z},$$

$$y = f\frac{Y}{Z}.$$

(C.1)

These equations are rather simple, compared to the equations for a 2D to 2D perspective projection described in chapter 1. This is because equations (C.1) use one global coordinate system related to the camera, whereas equations (A.1–A.2) use two separate coordinate systems. If an object point is known in a coordinate system $X'Y'Z'$, which is different than the coordinate system XYZ by a rotation R and translation T, then before equations (C.1) are applied, one has to express the coordinates of the point in the camera coordinate system. Let $V' = [X',Y',Z']^t$ be a column vector representing a point V in the object's coordinate system, $V = [X,Y,Z]^t$ be a column vector representing the point in the camera coordinate system, R be a 3×3 matrix and T be a 3×1 column vector $[t_1,t_2,t_3]^t$. Then,

$$V = R(V' - T). \tag{C.2}$$

The rotation matrix R has nine parameters, but only three of them are independent. These three parameters correspond to the three degrees of freedom for a rigid rotation in a 3D space. In other words, the elements r_{ij} of matrix R cannot be arbitrary numbers. Instead, they have to satisfy the following six constraints:

$$r_{11}^2 + r_{12}^2 + r_{13}^2 + 1, \ r_{11}r_{21} + r_{12}r_{22} + r_{13}r_{23} = 0,$$
$$r_{21}^2 + r_{22}^2 + r_{23}^2 + 1, \ r_{11}r_{31} + r_{12}r_{32} + r_{13}r_{33} = 0, \tag{C.3}$$
$$r_{31}^2 + r_{32}^2 + r_{33}^2 + 1, \ r_{21}r_{31} + r_{22}r_{32} + r_{23}r_{33} = 0.$$

In addition, the determinant of R must be equal to 1, not -1. A matrix that satisfies relations (C.3) is called an "orthonormal matrix," whose row vectors have length equal to one (i.e., they are normalized) and whose dot products are zero (i.e., they are orthogonal). Relations (C.3) could also be written for columns of a rotation matrix.

C.3 Homogeneous Coordinates for 3D to 2D Perspective Projection

The relations (C.1) in the previous section, representing a perspective projection, are nonlinear and thus cannot be represented as a matrix equation. This fact complicates mathematical treatment and makes it more difficult to use in machine vision applications. These relations can be rewritten by using homogeneous coordinates. Euclidean coordinates X,Y,Z can be rewritten as homogeneous coordinates as follows: $X^* = WX$, $Y^* = WY$, $Z^* = WZ$, $W^* = W$ (here, W can be set to 1, without restricting generality). It is easy to get Euclidean coordinates from homogeneous ones:

$$X = \frac{X^*}{W^*},$$
$$Y = \frac{Y^*}{W^*}, \tag{C.4}$$
$$Z = \frac{Z^*}{W^*}.$$

Similarly, we can introduce homogeneous coordinates on the image plane: $x^* = wx$, $y^* = wy$, $w^* = w$ (here, w cannot be set to an arbitrary value; instead, w is computed). Equation (C.1) can now be written in a matrix form. Let $v = [x^*,y^*,w^*]^t$, $V = [X^*,Y^*,Z^*,W^*]^t$. Let A be a 3×4 matrix. Then,

$$v = AV, \tag{C.5a}$$

where

$$A = \begin{bmatrix} 1 & 0 & 0 & 0 \\ 0 & 1 & 0 & 0 \\ 0 & 0 & 1/f & 0 \end{bmatrix}. \tag{C.5b}$$

The matrix equation (C.5a) represents three ordinary linear equations that are equivalent to the two nonlinear equations (C.1). To see the equivalence, we compute x from x^* and y from y^*:

$$x = \frac{x^*}{w^*} = \frac{X^*}{Z^*/f} = f\frac{X}{Z},$$
$$y = \frac{y^*}{w^*} = \frac{Y^*}{Z^*/f} = f\frac{Y}{Z}. \tag{C.6}$$

The main advantage of using homogeneous coordinates is that all transformations such as rigid motions and perspective projection can be done using matrix algebra, which corresponds to solving a set of linear equations, and then, at the end, the Euclidean coordinates on the image are easy to obtain by taking ratios x^*/w^* and y^*/w^*.

Once a perspective projection is expressed by a matrix equation, we can now combine transformations (C.1) and (C.2) (Mundy & Zisserman, 1992, chapter 23):

$$\begin{bmatrix} x^* \\ y^* \\ w^* \end{bmatrix} = \begin{bmatrix} 1 & 0 & 0 & 0 \\ 0 & 1 & 0 & 0 \\ 0 & 0 & 1/f & 0 \end{bmatrix} \begin{bmatrix} r_{11} & r_{12} & r_{13} & -R_1 \cdot T \\ r_{21} & r_{22} & r_{23} & -R_2 \cdot T \\ r_{31} & r_{32} & r_{33} & -R_3 \cdot T \\ 0 & 0 & 0 & 1 \end{bmatrix} \begin{bmatrix} X'^* \\ Y'^* \\ Z'^* \\ 1 \end{bmatrix}$$
$$= \begin{bmatrix} r_{11} & r_{12} & r_{13} & -R_1 \cdot T \\ r_{21} & r_{22} & r_{23} & -R_2 \cdot T \\ r_{31}/f & r_{32}/f & r_{33}/f & -R_3 \cdot T/f \end{bmatrix} \begin{bmatrix} X'^* \\ Y'^* \\ Z'^* \\ 1 \end{bmatrix}, \tag{C.7a}$$

where

$$R_1 \cdot T = r_{11}t_1 + r_{12}t_2 + r_{13}t_3,$$
$$R_2 \cdot T = r_{21}t_1 + r_{22}t_2 + r_{23}t_3, \tag{C.7b}$$
$$R_3 \cdot T = r_{31}t_1 + r_{32}t_2 + r_{33}t_3.$$

As already pointed out, equation (C.7a) is just another way to write equations (C.1–C.2). Given a camera with its coordinate system, an object represented in its own coordinate system, and the relation between the two coordinate systems, the formula (C.7a) allows the computation of a perspective image. The formula (C.7a) can be written in a more general way as $v = PV'$, where P is a 3×4 matrix:

$$
\begin{bmatrix} x^* \\ y^* \\ w^* \end{bmatrix} = \begin{bmatrix} p_{11} & p_{12} & p_{13} & p_{14} \\ p_{21} & p_{22} & p_{23} & p_{24} \\ p_{31} & p_{32} & p_{33} & p_{34} \end{bmatrix} \begin{bmatrix} X'^* \\ Y'^* \\ Z'^* \\ 1 \end{bmatrix}. \tag{C.8}
$$

If the matrix equation (C.8) is used to solve a problem involving perspective projection, then elements of matrix P are treated as independent. This corresponds to the case where the camera is not calibrated and its geometry is not known. As a result, perspective projection is represented by twelve parameters, from which eleven are independent (only eleven, not twelve, are independent because all elements of P can be divided by this element p_{kl} that is not zero; as a result, all elements of v on the left hand side of (C.8) will also be divided by p_{kl} without affecting the Euclidean coordinates (x,y) of v). This is the approach that Roberts (1965) took in his paper (see the introduction in chapter 3). Note that if elements of P are assumed to be unknown, then this matrix can always be postmultiplied by any 4×4 matrix without changing the result. Such multiplication corresponds to an arbitrary 3D projective transformation. This means that using homogeneous coordinates will not allow reconstructing Euclidean properties of an object, but only its projective properties. In particular, a 3D projectivity is characterized by $15df$. 3D shape is not changed by a rigid motion (3D rotation and translation) that is characterized by $6df$, or by size scaling ($1df$). It follows that a 3D projective transformation can change shape with $8df$, and the recognition system such as Roberts' will not be able to discriminate among those shapes. In other words, his method is subject to substantial shape ambiguity. This is the price one pays for the mathematical convenience of using linear equations. The human visual system does not do this. It uses the nonlinear equations and keeps shape ambiguity to a minimum.

Finally, a brief remark. Since equations (C.7) and (C.8) involve homogeneous coordinates, it is commonplace to call the transformation represented by these equations a "projective 3D to 2D transformation." This is misleading. As indicated more than once, a projective transformation is a one-to-one transformation. If a transformation is not a one-to-one mapping, it is not a group. Therefore, a 3D to 2D transformation is not a projectivity. For example, a set of non-coplanar points in 3D is always mapped to a set of coplanar points on a 2D image. However, coplanarity is a projective invariant. Because coplanarity is not preserved, this transformation is not a projectivity.

C.4 Calibrated versus Uncalibrated Cameras

In a calibrated camera, the geometry of the camera is known. This geometry is characterized by a distance f between the center of projection and the image plane, the coordinates of the principal point (x_o,y_o), that is a point of intersection of a line emanating from the center of projection and orthogonal to the image plane (usually $x_o = y_o = 0$), size of a sensor represented by scale factors (α_x,α_y) (usually $\alpha_x = \alpha_y = 1$), and a skew s of the sensor (usually $s = 0$). In order to explicitly represent all those parameters, the matrix A from equation (C.5b) representing a perspective projection takes the form (Hartley & Zisserman, 2003)

$$A = \begin{bmatrix} \alpha_x & s & x_o & 0 \\ 0 & \alpha_y & y_o & 0 \\ 0 & 0 & 1/f & 0 \end{bmatrix}. \tag{C.9}$$

If a camera is not calibrated, some or all of these parameters are unknown, and then a perspective projection is represented by a formula (C.8). And conversely, if homogeneous coordinates are used and a camera is represented by eleven independent parameters, as in equation (C.8), then the camera is treated as uncalibrated.

Existing psychophysical evidence shows that the human eye is a calibrated camera. In other words, the visual system "knows" the geometry of the eyeball and uses this information in achieving shape constancy. If the eye were an uncalibrated camera, we would perceive shapes in figure 3.10a and 3.10c as identical. That is, when an uncalibrated camera is used, all projectively equivalent shapes "look" the same. The fact that we achieve shape constancy in the case of perspective, but not projective transformations of shapes, shows that our eye is a calibrated camera.

C.5 Transformations and Invariants

Invariants have been known in mathematics for a long time. An "invariant" refers to a feature that does not change under some set of transformations (Klein, 1939). In geometry, invariants have received special status as explained by Felix Klein in an inaugural talk when he accepted a position at the University of Erlangen in 1872. Klein stated that the study of geometry should be organized around the concept of groups of transformations and their invariants (since then this claim has been called an *"Erlanger Programm"*). A set of transformations is called a "group" when it satisfies four axioms. A set of translations on a plane will be used to introduce these axioms. Translations form a group because, first, there is a zero translation (called an "identity" translation); second, for each translation, there is always another translation, called an "inverse," so if one of these translations is followed by the other, the result (called a "product" or "composition") is an identity translation; third, a composition of any two translations is a translation (a property called "closure"); and fourth, in a sequence of three translations performed one after another, the final result does not depend on whether (i) the composition of the first two is followed by the third or (ii) the first is followed by the composition of the last two (a property called "associativity").

There are several main groups of geometrical transformations: namely, rigid motion, similarity (both called Euclidean groups), affine, projectivity, and topology. Some of those groups are of interest in shape perception either because they can be used to describe shape (similarity group) or because they are relevant in the context of image formation in the human eye (affine and projective). Once a good mathematical treatment of both is at hand, one can formulate a theory of perception of shapes based on the information present in retinal images.

"Rigid motion" refers to translations and rotations (see figure C.1). 2D rigid motion (rigid motion on a plane) corresponds to a rotation by an angle φ and translation by a vector (t_x, t_y):

$$x' = x\cos\varphi - y\sin\varphi + t_x,$$
$$y' = x\sin\varphi + y\cos\varphi + t_y. \qquad (C.10)$$

Rigid motion is characterized by *3df*. Euclidean distance is invariant under rigid motion. Obviously, moving an object or a figure around in a rigid fashion does not change any distances within the object.

If, in addition to rigid motion, one allows uniform-size scaling, a similarity group is formed (figure C.2). 2D similarity group is represented by the following formulas:

$$x' = k(x\cos\varphi - y\sin\varphi + t_x),$$
$$y' = k(x\sin\varphi + y\cos\varphi + t_y). \qquad (C.11)$$

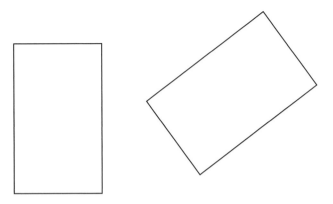

Figure C.1
2D Euclidean transformation (rigid motion).

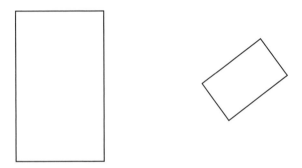

Figure C.2
2D similarity transformation.

Similarity transformation is characterized by 4*df*. Here, distance is no longer invariant, but the size of an angle and the ratio of distances are invariant. It is important to note that the similarity group is usually used to define shape. That is, shape has usually been defined as those geometrical aspects of an object or a figure that do not change under the similarity group of transformations. This definition is too narrow because some objects would be classified as having the same shape, even though one cannot be obtained by a similarity transformation of the other. An example would be a table in which one drills a small hole. The hole, which is a nontopological transformation, cannot be undone by a rigid motion plus size scaling.

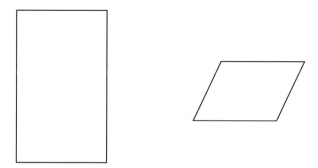

Figure C.3
2D affine transformation.

Consider next the affine group. This is the smallest group that is relevant to the process of image formation in the human eye. The affine group is obtained when one allows a uniform stretch of an object or a figure in an arbitrary direction, in addition to rigid motion and size scaling (figure C.3). 2D affine group is represented by the following formulas:

$$x' = ax + by + c,$$
$$y' = dx + ey + f.$$
(C.12)

A direction in a plane requires one parameter (an angle), and the magnitude of stretch requires another. It follows that a 2D affine transformation has 6*df* as is clear from equation (C.12). Distances and angles are not invariant anymore, but the ratio of lengths of two parallel line segments is an affine invariant. Another 2D affine invariant is the ratio of areas of two corresponding regions specified by four points on a plane. In a 3D affine transformation, the corresponding invariant is defined as a ratio of two volumes specified by five points. In the context of image formation in the eye or a camera, a 2D affine group is more relevant than a 3D affine group. A 2D affine transformation can be used as an approximation of a projection of planar figures to the retinal or camera image. This approximation is good when the projecting lines are approximately parallel. This happens when the size of a planar figure is small as compared to the viewing distance. It follows that affine invariants could provide an explanation of shape constancy in the case of small figures. For large figures, however, a parallel projection is not a good approximation to a perspective projection, which means that affine invariants cannot provide a full explanation of

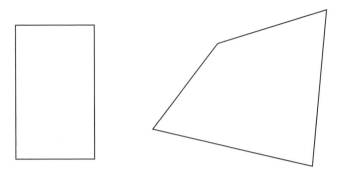

Figure C.4
2D projective transformation.

human shape perception. A 3D affine group is relevant when a parallel projection of a 3D space to two images is considered (e.g., Koenderink & van Doorn, 1991).

When perspective projections are allowed, one obtains a projective group (figure C.4). Perspective projections are of special interest here because they describe the formation of the retinal image. In particular, a projective transformation is a composition (product) of two or more perspective projections. And conversely, any projective transformation can be represented by a product of at most two perspective projections (relation between perspective and projective transformation is presented in section C.7). Formulas for a 2D projectivity are presented in appendix A, section A.2. Using homogeneous coordinates x^*,y^*,w^* and x'^*,y'^*,w'^*, a 2D projectivity is represented by the following matrix equation:

$$\begin{bmatrix} x'^* \\ y'^* \\ w'^* \end{bmatrix} = \begin{bmatrix} a & b & c \\ d & e & f \\ g & h & i \end{bmatrix} \begin{bmatrix} x^* \\ y^* \\ w^* \end{bmatrix}. \tag{C.13}$$

Euclidean coordinates on each plane are obtained by taking ratios: $x = x^*/w^*$, $y = y^*/w^*$, $x' = x'^*/w'^*$, $y' = y'^*/w'^*$. By taking these ratios, it is easy to verify the equivalence of equations (C.13) and (A.5).

Finally, consider the group of topological transformations. The topological group includes all continuous transformations. Topological transformations of a plane are usually illustrated by a rubber sheath that can be stretched arbitrarily without tearing or cutting it. The topological group has only a few invariants. For example, two intersecting lines remain intersecting after a topological transformation.

The five groups described above form a hierarchy with rigid motion being smallest (least general) and topology being largest (most general). Topology has the fewest invariants, and rigid motion has the most invariants. A property that is preserved in a larger group is also preserved in a smaller group.

C.6   Projective Invariants in Machine Vision

Duda and Hart (1973) were the first to discuss projective invariants in the context of computer vision. Their book, which provides a brief tutorial about projective invariants, includes a couple of simple examples. However, with the exception of this book, the machine vision community did not pay attention to projective invariants until 1988. That year, Isaac Weiss published his first paper on this important topic (Weiss, 1988a). He indicated which invariants can be applied to point sets and which to smooth curves. Invariants that can be applied to point sets are easier to use, and, therefore, they received more attention (see Weiss, 1993, for a review). Note that point sets are directly related to polygons. Figure 3.7 in section 3.3.2 illustrated the application of the cross ratio of four areas to a simple polygon. This example also illustrated limitations of projective invariants as an explanation of shape constancy. Specifically, the visual system can deal effectively with a perspective transformation, including small distortions of a perspective transformation, but not with an arbitrary projective transformation.

Using cross ratios of four areas in order to verify projective equivalence is fairly easy, as long as the areas are polygons because polygons have distinctive points for which the correspondence is easy to establish. In the case of smoothly curved figures that do not have distinctive points, one has to use differential or integral projective invariants (Weiss, 1988a, 1993; Mundy & Zisserman, 1992). From these two types of invariants, integral invariants (such as moments) are useless with images of real scenes because in the presence of occlusions such invariants cannot be computed (Rothwell, 1995). Differential invariants also have their problems because they are very sensitive to noise in the camera image. One way to avoid problems inherent in integral and differential invariants in the case of smooth curves is to identify characteristic points such as "concavity entrance" (Lamdan, Schwartz, & Wolfson, 1988; Rothwell, 1995), which then can be used to compute cross ratios, or to represent the entire curve in an invariant (canonical) form.

Invariants may be applied to a part of an object (or a figure), but they must not include points or features that do not belong to the object of interest. Otherwise, the value of the invariant will be incorrect. It follows that the application of invariants must be preceded by establishing figure–ground organization.

Despite the fact that the formulation of projective geometry and projective invariants was motivated by the properties of perspective projection, they cannot be applied to the most interesting case of perception of 3D objects for the simple reason that the perspective transformation from a 3D space to a 2D image is not a group. A projective transformation is only possible between spaces of identical dimensions: between two lines, between two planes, or between two 3D spaces. However, no projective transformation exists between a 3D space and a plane because this is not a one-to-one mapping. It follows that group axioms are violated: There is no identity transformation, there is no unique inverse, and the composition (product) does not exist. These violations of group axioms must have been obvious to mathematicians, but the first publication describing the implications of these violations appeared only in 1990 (Burns et al., 1990). Burns et al. stated and proved that there is no general case invariant for the 3D to 2D projection. By general case, it was meant the case of an arbitrary set of points in 3D with no restriction on the type of 3D structures or their 3D orientation. The gist of the proof involves a sequence of sets of points in 3D such that each pair of sets from this sequence is different from one another with respect to one point only. Since it is always possible to find a center of projection such that two different points in 3D map to the same point on a 2D image, it follows that these two sets are equivalent under 3D to 2D mapping. For N points, one simply needs N sets of points to show that any set of N points is equivalent to any other set of N points under 3D to 2D projection. Therefore, if there is an invariant of such a mapping, it would be a trivial one because its value would be identical for all sets of N points. It follows that conventional invariants cannot be applied to arbitrary 3D objects, but only to planar or approximately planar figures.

However, even if one is willing to work with planar figures, projective invariants may not accomplish what one expects. Projective invariants are quite sensitive to visual noise (Astrom, 1995). This implies that even though a projective invariant can be computed, its value may be difficult to interpret. This is the reason why affine invariants received more attention than projective invariants (Mundy & Zisserman, 1992; Mundy et al., 1993). But affine invariants can only be applied to cases where affine transformation is a good approximation to a perspective transformation. Such cases involve figures whose size is small compared to the viewing distance or, more generally, cases in which the range in depth of the slanted figure is small relative to the viewing distance.

An interesting alternative is to work with perspective projection itself, despite the fact that perspective transformations do not form a group. Perspective projection is important for at least two reasons: First, it is a better model of retinal image formation, and second, it provides the maximal number of constraints for a vision geometry. It will be shown that the perspective model leads to powerful methods for shape reconstruction and recognition, involving model-based invariants and a priori constraints. These aspects of shape perception dominate the second half of this book. Next, the details of the perspective model will be described.

C.7 Projectivity versus Perspectivity

We already know that 2D perspectivity differs from 2D projectivity in that some terms are absent in the formulas for the former (appendix A, sections A.1–A.2). Let's examine the relation between perspectivity and projectivity for the 1D case. The following equations represent a perspectivity (C.14a) and a projectivity (C.14b) in 1D:

$$x' = \frac{ax}{cx + d}, \tag{C.14a}$$

$$x' = \frac{ax + b}{cx + d}. \tag{C.14b}$$

Perspectivity has fewer degrees of freedom. In equation (C.14a), where the origin of x is mapped onto the origin of x', there are only three parameters, two of which are independent. Projectivity (equation C.14b) has four parameters, three of which are independent. It should be clear by looking at these equations that a 1D projectivity corresponds to a perspectivity followed by a translation (see figure C.5). In general, a 1D projectivity can be produced by applying 1D perspectivity more than once. A product of

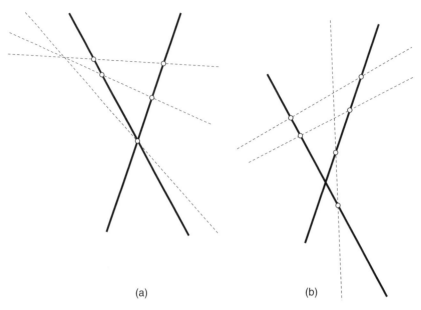

(a)   (b)

Figure C.5
Perspectivity versus projectivity between lines. In (a), the projecting lines intersect at a single point, which is the center of perspective projection. In (b), the points on one line were translated. Now, the projecting lines do not intersect at a single point. This means that the mapping in (b) is not a perspective projection, although it is a projectivity.

two different perspectivities, one between line L_1 and L_2 and another between L_2 and L_3, is itself a perspectivity between L_1 and L_3 if all three lines intersect at a common point P that maps onto itself. This is illustrated in figure C.6. A proof of this statement follows from two facts: (i) A 1D projectivity is uniquely defined by a projection of three points, and (ii) two different projecting lines, representing the projection of the non-intersection points, always intersect or are parallel. The intersection point of these two projecting lines (this point may lie at infinity) is the center of perspective projection. The third projecting line, which maps P onto itself, can have an arbitrary orientation and, in particular, can also go through this center of perspective projection. Thus, the projectivity between L_1 and L_3 is a perspective projection.

By analogy, a 2D projectivity (projectivity between two planes) is a 2D perspectivity followed by a 2D translation and 2D rotation, and a product

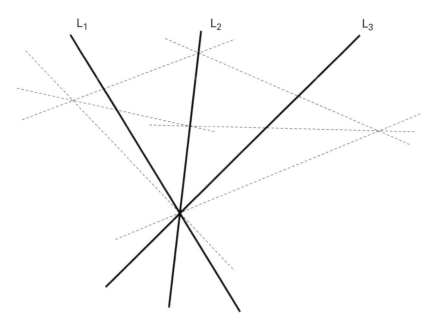

Figure C.6
Product of a perspectivity between L_1 and L_2, and between L_2 and L_3, is also a perspectivity between L_1 and L_3 (after Pizlo, 1994).

of two perspectivities is itself a perspectivity if the three planes involved in this product intersect at a common line that maps onto itself. This implies that any projective transformation of a planar figure can be produced on a camera image, but the position, size, and orientation of the image may not conform to the rules of perspective projection. Consider an example. Figure C.7 shows three polygons. When the polygon in (b) is viewed from a distance five times larger than the size of the figure, it looks like a slanted (a). However, (c) does not look like a slanted (a) even though (c) is a perspective image of (a). The image in (c) was produced by placing the camera very close to the figure, with its visual axis away from the figure. Thus, in order for (c) to produce a valid perspective image of (a) in the observer's eye, the observer would have to fixate at the cross at a viewing distance equal to six tenths of the distance between the cross and the center of the polygon in (c).[2] This example illustrates several important things. First, the visual system "knows" the difference between a perspective projection and a projective transformation. This makes sense because

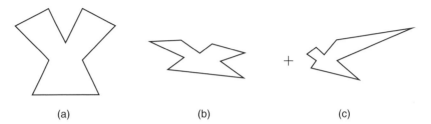

(a)   (b)   (c)

Figure C.7
Perspective images of a polygon in (a). The plane of the figure should be orthogonal
to the line of sight. When (b) is viewed from a distance that is five times larger than
the diameter of the figure, the retinal image of (b) is a perspective image of a slanted
(a) with tilt 80 deg and slant 70 deg. The retinal image of (c) is a perspective image
of a slanted (a) when the reader fixates at the cross from a distance equal to six
tenths of the distance between the center of the polygon and the fixation cross
(practical suggestion: project (c) on a large screen). Otherwise, the retinal image of
(c) is a projective image of (a).

when one is viewing actual scenes, the retinal image in the observer's eye
is not an arbitrary projective image. It is always a perspective image.
Second, the visual system knows the positions of the fovea and the focal
point. If it didn't, then we wouldn't be able to tell the difference between
figure C.7b and C.7c. Recall that these aspects of projective geometry were
briefly discussed in chapter 2 in the context of Perkins' contributions. His
results made it possible to conclude that the visual system knows the
geometry of the eyeball, as well as the rules of perspective projection.
Finally, and most importantly, the example in figure C.7 shows that understanding the geometry of image formation is useful in understanding shape
perception. We will, therefore, explore the geometry of image formation
in some more detail in the subsequent sections.

Because perspective projection is not a group, it does not have its own
invariants. Invariants of a perspective projection are also invariants of the
smallest group generated by perspective projections, which is the projective group. However, we already know that projective invariants cannot
explain shape constancy (e.g., figures 3.10 and C.7). We can conclude that
human shape constancy involves invariants of transformations that are
outside the *Erlanger Programm*. Before these invariants are described, a
model of image formation has to be discussed.

C.8 Model of Image Formation

A perspective image in the human eye or camera is formed by light rays. In an optically uniform medium, such as air, light rays are straight lines. If we don't count optical distortions in the human eye, the light rays intersect at a single point called the "nodal point," and this point is the center of perspective projection. This is why geometrical perspective is used as a model of image formation. Note, however, that light is propagated in one direction at a time, and this fact has several implications for image formation in the human eye or a camera, even though these implications do not apply to geometrical perspective. One such implication is that the object and its image are always on opposite sides of the center of perspective projection. This, in turn, implies that if an infinitely large plane "out there" is considered an object, only one half of this plane will produce an image (Pizlo, Rosenfeld, & Weiss, 1997a, b). Next, the order of three points on the line is preserved in optical perspective, and convexity of a figure is preserved, as well. None of these properties exist in geometrical perspective projection or in a projective geometry.

Next, in the human eye, the center of projection is fixed relative to the retina. Specifically, the distance to the center of projection from the retina (approximately equal to the focal distance) is constant. Furthermore, the point of intersection (the center of fovea) of the retina with the line emanating from the center of projection and orthogonal to the retina is fixed in the retinal coordinate system. Neither the focal distance nor the fovea is fixed in an uncalibrated camera, which is used as a model of projective transformation. Fixing the focal distance does not make sense in projective geometry because Euclidean distance does not exist in this geometry. Projective geometry cannot use properties from more specific geometries. Doing so would result in the group structure of geometry being destroyed. And this is the main point here: Image formation in the human eye in particular, and spatial vision in general, does not conform to the formalism of group theory.

A model that represents all important aspects of image formation in the human eye and a camera was described by Pizlo, Rosenfeld, and Weiss (1997a) and was called a "fixed center directional perspective" (FCDP). In the case of planar figures, FCDP is represented by equations given in appendix A, section A.1. For a given position, orientation, and size of the retinal image, FCDP can change a 2D shape with $2df$ corresponding to slant and tilt. By allowing the retinal position, orientation, and size to change, one can reproduce all 2D projective transformations of shape (more specifically, those projective transformations that do not involve points behind the retina). Recall that 2D projectivity can change a shape with $4df$. This fact leads to a common misconception about the relation between 2D projectivity and image formation in the human eye. The fact that all 2D projective transformations of a *shape* can be reproduced on the retina does not imply that all 2D projective transformations of a *figure* can be reproduced on the retina. The reason is that image formation in the human eye has fewer degrees of freedom than 2D projectivity. This means that although all four-dimensional transformations of a 2D shape can be produced on the retina, the resulting retinal images cannot have arbitrary sizes, orientations, and positions. Size, orientation, and position are not free parameters in image formation.

FCDP was used for years in the photogrammetry literature, and later on in computer vision (see Haralick & Shapiro, 1993, for a review). The methods that use FCDP were developed in order to determine which aspects of 3D scenes can be computed from real camera images. The case of visual reconstruction from two or more camera images was discussed in section 3.2. Here, we will concentrate on the case of a single image. The first invariants of FCDP for the case of a single image of a planar figure were formulated in 1990 (Pizlo & Rosenfeld, 1990, 1992) and then tested in psychophysical experiments (Pizlo, 1994). These invariants, which are precursors of model-based invariants for 3D objects, allow one to recognize a 2D shape from a single retinal image (see the next section). Specifically, *these invariants allow one to recognize similarity structure of a 2D figure, characterized by angles and ratios of distances, despite projective distortions of the figure that are present in the retinal image.* Recall that projective distortions change angles and ratios of distances. This is a very important result. Recognition of similarity properties based on images in which these properties have been changed projectively is not possible in conventional geometry that is based on group structure. In conventional geometry, once a given feature is changed by a transformation, it cannot be reconstructed or recognized because more general groups do not have access to properties from less general ones. Recognition of properties of a smaller group despite distortions produced by transformations from a larger group is possible only if these transformations themselves do not form a group. To be precise, under some conditions, which were referred to in chapter 1 as "shape ambiguity," application of invariants of FCDP leads to failure of shape recognition. But so does human shape recognition as shown by Thouless (1931a, b). Such failures are probably not critical for the case of shape perception in everyday life because shape ambiguity happens very rarely (with a probability of zero).[3]

C.9   Invariants of Perspective Projection

First, invariants of 2D to 2D perspective projection are presented, and then invariants of 3D to 2D perspective projection are presented.

C.9.1   2D Invariants

Consider the task of recognizing a planar shape S from a single-perspective image I(S) obtained with a tilt τ_I, slant σ_I, and viewing distance C_I (see appendix A, section A.1) using a calibrated camera. This task is called "shape constancy" (see chapter 1). It can be solved, at least in principle, by performing a search through all slants, tilts, and viewing distances. Specifically, we can take S and compute its perspective images for all triplets of values τ, σ, and C. We then compare all these images to I(S) and check whether any of them are identical to I(S). If such an image can be found, one can conclude that I(S) has been produced by S (i.e., S has been recognized based on I(S)). Otherwise, the image I(S) could not have been produced by S. One can simplify the search if inverse perspective images of I(S) are computed because an inverse perspective projection with a calibrated camera affects a planar shape with only two, not three degrees of freedom, slant, and tilt. Thus, we take I(S) and compute its inverse perspective images for all pairs of values τ and σ. We then compare these images to S and check whether any of them are identical to S.

Assume that tilt τ is known but slant σ is not known. Pizlo and Rosenfeld (1992) showed that the search for slant can be eliminated by using perspective invariants. Consider the Ψ function, which characterizes a contour of a 2D figure. The Ψ function is a standard tool in computer vision (see Ballard & Brown, 1982). To plot this function, one starts at a point on the contour and plots the orientation of the tangent line at this point. Then, one moves along the contour and plots the orientation of the tangent as a function of the distance from the starting point. An example is shown

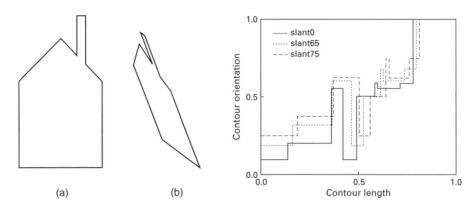

Figure C.8
A planar shape (a), its perspective image (b), and the corresponding ψ functions (from Pizlo & Salach-Golyska, 1995).

in figure C.8. If we apply inverse perspective transformations with tilt τ and with several slants σ_i to a planar shape, the corresponding Ψ functions will form a family that has two important characteristics: (i) The corresponding points of the functions are approximately collinear (see figure C.8), and (ii) for any pair of the Ψ functions, Ψ_j and Ψ_k, representing the inverse perspective images of a given retinal shape with slants σ_j and σ_k, a ratio of distances between the corresponding points of the functions is approximately constant and equal for all points around the contour:

$$\frac{\Psi_j - \Psi_0}{\Psi_k - \Psi_0} \approx constant = \frac{\sigma_j^2}{\sigma_k^2}, \tag{C.15}$$

where Ψ_0 characterizes the perspective image whose shape is to be recognized.

How can those two invariant properties be used in solving the shape constancy task? Let A be a perspective image whose shape is to be recognized, and B a reference figure whose shape is known. Specifically, we assume that Ψ_B is known when B was in the frontal plane (slant zero). It is hypothesized that the figure A was obtained by slanting B with a known tilt τ_B and unknown slant σ_B. We begin with constructing Ψ_A and then computing an inverse perspective projection of A with tilt τ_B and slant σ_C. Slant σ_C may be arbitrary, although the approximation works well when this slant is between 60 and 70 deg. We then construct Ψ_C. Shape A is a valid perspective image of B *if and only if* Ψ_A, Ψ_B, and Ψ_C satisfy the two properties (i) and (ii). Specifically, in criterion (C.15), we put $\Psi_0 = \Psi_A$, $\Psi_j = \Psi_B$, and $\Psi_k = \Psi_C$. If the criterion (C.15) is satisfied for all (or most) points on the contour, one can conclude that A is an image of B and the unknown slant σ_B can be estimated from the constant in (C.15).

If tilt τ_B is unknown, then one has to try several tilts (see Pizlo & Rosenfeld, 1992). The search for tilt can be simplified by using affine invariants. Recall that 2D affine transformation can be used as an approximation to perspective projection. Even if the approximation is not perfect, the least squares estimators can be obtained and then an estimate of tilt can be derived from these estimates. Affine transformation is identical for tilts τ and $\tau + 180$ deg, which means that two values of tilt would have to be tried after the tilt is estimated from affine approximation. One could try to apply other methods to eliminate the search for tilt entirely, but this may not be justified from a perceptual point of view. Specifically, Pizlo (1994) showed that uncertainty about tilt harms shape constancy performance, which suggests that the human visual system does perform some search for the tilt value.

C.9.2   3D Invariants

The question posed by Pizlo and Loubier (2000) was how to modify Roberts' recognition method so that it can be applied to the case of a calibrated camera. The key observation made by Pizlo and Loubier was that the criterion for the alignment of an object with its retinal image is computationally simpler when object points are compared to projecting planes, rather than lines. Planes in 3D have simpler parametric representations than lines. As a result, a squared distance of a point from a plane is a quadratic function of the unknown parameters representing the position and orientation of the 3D object relative to the camera. It follows that the best alignment of the object with the image, represented by the sum of squared distances of the object points from the corresponding projecting planes, has a closed form solution. More exactly, the closed form solution can be obtained only when one allows an arbitrary 3D affine transformation of the object, not just a 3D rigid motion. Once the parameters of the 3D affine transformation are estimated, it can be verified whether this transformation satisfies (approximately) constraints represented by the rigid motion (the 3×3 matrix must be orthonormal, with a positive determinant—see equation C.3).

These 3D perspective invariants have been tested in simulations. However, they have not been tested yet as a model of human shape constancy.

C.10   3D Model-Based Projective Invariants

Rothwell (1995) described model-based invariants for several classes of objects. Consider solids of revolution first. All intersections of a rotationally symmetrical object with planes orthogonal to its axis of symmetry are circles. A simple example of a solid of revolution is a circular cylinder. A perspective image of a solid of revolution is a symmetrical figure (with mirror symmetry) only in a special case when the line of sight intersects the axis of symmetry (figure C.9a). This fact follows from the symmetry of the object and symmetry of perspective projection itself. Under such viewing conditions, it is easy to find the symmetry axis of the image, as well as features of the image that are mirror symmetrical, such as external and internal bitangent lines (Rothwell, 1995, p. 198). Bitangent lines are straight lines that are tangent to the contours of the image at two points. Because of symmetry of the image, corresponding bitangent lines are mirror symmetrical, and so they intersect at points on the symmetry axis. These points can be used to compute a conventional cross ratio of four collinear points, which

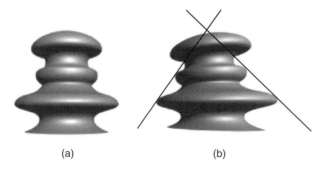

(a)   (b)

Figure C.9
An image of a solid of revolution when the line of sight intersected the axis of symmetry (a) and when the line of sight was away from the axis of symmetry (b). A pair of bitangent lines are shown. Image (b) is a 2D projective transformation of image (a) (produced using 3DS Max/Autodesk).

is a projective invariant. Now, when the line of sight does not intersect the axis of symmetry of the solid of revolution, then the perspective image is no longer symmetrical (figure C.9b). However, it is easy to see that this image is a 2D projective transformation of the image produced when the line of sight does intersect the axis of symmetry of the object (Kanatani, 1988). Since straight lines and tangent points are projective invariants, it follows that bitangent lines still intersect at the image of the axis of symmetry of the object and the cross ratio computed from these points is invariant in any perspective image of a given solid of revolution.

When an object is bilaterally symmetrical (i.e., it has mirror symmetry), then another method is used. A perspective image of a symmetrical object can be treated as two perspective images of an asymmetrical object (i.e., of one half of the object). Then, any of the standard algorithms for reconstructing an object from two perspective images can be applied to the two parts of the image representing the two halves of the symmetrical object.[4] If the camera is calibrated, Longuet-Higgins' (1981) algorithm (or any of its variants) can be used for reconstructing a Euclidean structure of the object. If the camera is uncalibrated, a projective structure of the object can be computed (see Rothwell, 1995, for a review). If the image is a result of a parallel, rather than perspective, projection, then an affine structure can be computed by using Koenderink and van Doorn's (1991) method.

Next, consider model-based invariants for polyhedra. It is important to point out right away that these invariants can be applied only to those polyhedra whose projective structure can be reconstructed by the method introduced by Sugihara (1986) and described in the beginning of chapter 3. Thus, model-based projective invariants do not provide a tighter specification of the family of objects, compared to Sugihara's method. In fact, since Rothwell's method is designed to compute 3D projective invariants, the family of shapes is larger than when a direct reconstruction is performed with a calibrated camera. In a sense, model-based projective invariants are even more qualitative than Sugihara's reconstruction method. Rothwell considered polyhedra where all vertices were trihedral. That is, each vertex was an intersection of three planar faces. This restriction has been used quite commonly in machine vision literature, although it is not clear how well this restriction is satisfied by real objects. Figure C.10 shows a polyhedron that does not look unnatural but has several vertices that

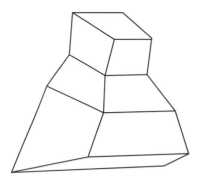

Figure C.10
A polyhedron where not all vertices are trihedral.

violate the trihedral assumption. By using homogeneous coordinates, Rothwell was able to write all relations describing faces of the polyhedron, perspective projection for uncalibrated camera, and vertices in the image using linear equations. It is then easy to eliminate unknown parameters and form invariants (Rothwell, 1995, pp. 200–5). Again, 3D projective invariants are insensitive to 3D projective transformation, which has 15df. 3D rigid motions (translations and rotations) and overall size scaling, which do not change 3D shape, are characterized by only 7df. It follows that 3D projective invariants are insensitive to changes of shape with 8df. This means that quite different shapes may be confused by a method based on projective invariants. A calibrated camera specifies a shape of a polyhedron up to a subset of 3D projective transformations with only 3df, as demonstrated by Sugihara (see also section C.11 in this appendix). This subset is quite small, and it contains only those 3D shapes that are perspectively, not projectively, equivalent. It follows that 3D projective invariants provide less information about shape than the shape reconstruction method described by Sugihara (1986).

C.11 Perspective Reconstruction of Polyhedra

Consider a perspective image of a hexahedron with quadrilateral faces. In particular, assume that all eight vertices and all twelve edges are shown in the image, as if the object were transparent (hidden points are not removed from the image). For simplicity of this analysis, but without restricting generality, assume that this hexahedron has the shape of a cube (figure

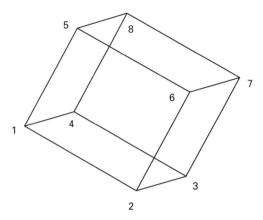

Figure C.11
The shape of a hexahedron like the one shown can be changed with 3*df* without changing its perspective image.

C.11). We want to establish the number of degrees of freedom with which the shape of the object "out there" could be changed so that (i) its image will still be identical with the given image and (ii) the object itself will be a polyhedron (planar faces stay planar). Constraint (i) is enforced by allowing each of the eight vertices to move along the projecting lines that emanate from the center of projection of the perspective camera (the projecting lines are not shown in figure C.11). This means that there are at most 8*df*. Since multiplying the 3D Euclidean coordinates of all vertices by the same number changes the size but not the shape of the object, the position of one vertex (say vertex 1) can be fixed at an arbitrary point on its projecting line without restricting generality. Vertices 2 and 3 can be moved arbitrarily along their projecting lines. This gives 2*df*. Vertex 4 is not independent because it must satisfy the planarity of the contour 1,2,3,4 and is obtained as an intersection of plane 1,2,3 and the projecting line of vertex 4. Vertex 5 can be moved arbitrarily on its projecting line. This increases the number of degrees of freedom to three. It is easy to check that the remaining vertices, 6, 7, and 8, are not independent. Vertex 6 is obtained as an intersection of plane 1,2,5 and the projecting line of vertex 6. Next, vertex 7 is obtained as an intersection of plane 2,3,6 and the projecting line of vertex 7, and vertex 8 is obtained as an intersection of plane 5,6,7 and the projecting line of vertex 8. Thus, when reconstructing a hexahedron having quadrilateral faces from its single-perspective image using a calibrated camera, the family of possible shapes is characterized by three parameters. This result is analogous to the result presented by Sugihara (1986). For more complex polyhedra, the number of degrees of freedom may be greater. However, the complexity of the object is not the primary factor. For example, in the case of the polyhedron in figure C.10, which is more complex than a cube, the number of degrees of freedom is only three, the same as for a cube.

Next, we will arrive at the three-parameter family of shape transformations by trying all 3D projective transformations of an object that leave the object's *perspective* image intact (Chan et al., 2006). Note that this family cannot be larger than the family established in the previous paragraph, because 3D projective transformations preserve coplanarity of points. Using the notation from section C.3 in this appendix, the 3D to 2D perspective projection can be represented by the following equation:

$$\begin{bmatrix} x^* \\ y^* \\ w^* \end{bmatrix} = \begin{bmatrix} 1 & 0 & 0 & 0 \\ 0 & 1 & 0 & 0 \\ 0 & 0 & 1/f & 0 \end{bmatrix} \begin{bmatrix} X^* \\ Y^* \\ Z^* \\ 1 \end{bmatrix}. \tag{C.16}$$

The left-hand side represents the image point using homogeneous coordinates, and the column vector on the right-hand side represents an object point using homogeneous coordinates. The matrix on the right-hand side represents a perspective projection by a calibrated camera. A 3D projective transformation is represented by a 4×4 matrix K. Now, we want to projectively transform an object point so that its image stays the same. This is equivalent to the following:

$$\begin{bmatrix} x^* \\ y^* \\ w^* \end{bmatrix} = \begin{bmatrix} 1 & 0 & 0 & 0 \\ 0 & 1 & 0 & 0 \\ 0 & 0 & 1/f & 0 \end{bmatrix} \begin{bmatrix} k_{11} & k_{12} & k_{13} & k_{14} \\ k_{21} & k_{22} & k_{23} & k_{24} \\ k_{31} & k_{32} & k_{33} & k_{34} \\ k_{41} & k_{42} & k_{43} & k_{44} \end{bmatrix} \begin{bmatrix} X^* \\ Y^* \\ Z^* \\ 1 \end{bmatrix}. \tag{C.17}$$

The left-hand sides in (C.16) and (C.17) are assumed to be equal because the retinal image does not change. Hence, the right-hand sides are equal:

$$\begin{bmatrix} 1 & 0 & 0 & 0 \\ 0 & 1 & 0 & 0 \\ 0 & 0 & 1/f & 0 \end{bmatrix} \begin{bmatrix} X^* \\ Y^* \\ Z^* \\ 1 \end{bmatrix} = \begin{bmatrix} 1 & 0 & 0 & 0 \\ 0 & 1 & 0 & 0 \\ 0 & 0 & 1/f & 0 \end{bmatrix} \begin{bmatrix} k_{11} & k_{12} & k_{13} & k_{14} \\ k_{21} & k_{22} & k_{23} & k_{24} \\ k_{31} & k_{32} & k_{33} & k_{34} \\ k_{41} & k_{42} & k_{43} & k_{44} \end{bmatrix} \begin{bmatrix} X^* \\ Y^* \\ Z^* \\ 1 \end{bmatrix}. \tag{C.18}$$

From (C.18) it follows that

$$\begin{bmatrix} 1 & 0 & 0 & 0 \\ 0 & 1 & 0 & 0 \\ 0 & 0 & 1/f & 0 \end{bmatrix} = \begin{bmatrix} 1 & 0 & 0 & 0 \\ 0 & 1 & 0 & 0 \\ 0 & 0 & 1/f & 0 \end{bmatrix} \begin{bmatrix} k_{11} & k_{12} & k_{13} & k_{14} \\ k_{21} & k_{22} & k_{23} & k_{24} \\ k_{31} & k_{32} & k_{33} & k_{34} \\ k_{41} & k_{42} & k_{43} & k_{44} \end{bmatrix}. \tag{C.19}$$

Hence,

$$\begin{bmatrix} 1 & 0 & 0 & 0 \\ 0 & 1 & 0 & 0 \\ 0 & 0 & 1/f & 0 \end{bmatrix} = \begin{bmatrix} k_{11} & k_{12} & k_{13} & k_{14} \\ k_{21} & k_{22} & k_{23} & k_{24} \\ k_{31}/f & k_{32}/f & k_{33}/f & k_{34}/f \end{bmatrix}. \tag{C.20}$$

It is easy to see that (C.20) is satisfied when K has the following form:

$$K = \begin{bmatrix} 1 & 0 & 0 & 0 \\ 0 & 1 & 0 & 0 \\ 0 & 0 & 1 & 0 \\ k_{41} & k_{42} & k_{43} & k_{44} \end{bmatrix}. \tag{C.21}$$

It follows from (C.21) that there are only $4df$ with which a 3D object can be projectively transformed without changing its perspective image. It is easy to see that k_{44} changes the size of a 3D object only and can be set to one. Thus, there are only $3df$ with which the shape of a 3D object can be projectively changed without changing its perspective image. This agrees with Sugihara's (1986) analysis for parallel projection of simple polyhedra (theorem 5.2, p. 95). It follows, that when the family of the reconstructed polyhedron is characterized by only $3df$ (like in the case of hexahedrons with quadrilateral faces), this family is a subset of all 3D projective transformations. This shows (again) that the model-based invariants of Rothwell (1995) do not provide a more restricted family of shapes than Sugihara's (1986) method. In fact, the converse is true because model-based projective invariants provide a family of 3D shapes that are not necessarily consistent with a given *perspective* image.

C.12   Regularization Solution to a Circle Problem

Let Y represent the data as obtained by visual receptors (figure 3.13c) and X the reconstructed (perceived) curve. Let $\|Y_i - X\|$ be the shortest distance between a given data point and the curve, and $\kappa(s)$ the curvature of X at a point specified by an arc length s (Hilbert & Cohn-Vossen, 1952). The reconstructed curve is the one that minimizes the following cost function:

$$E(X) = \|Y - X\|^2 + \lambda \|d\kappa/ds\|^2. \tag{C.22}$$

The first term on the right-hand side represents the sum of squared distances of points from the reconstructed curve, and the second term represents an integral of the squared first derivative of curvature along the entire contour of the curve. The first derivative of curvature, $d\kappa/ds$, is zero when the curvature is constant. It follows that the cost function (C.22) favors curves that are as circular (or as straight) as possible. When λ is close to zero, then the reconstructed curve will go through all data points. When λ goes to infinity, the reconstructed curve will be circular.

It has been argued that better results are obtained when compactness, rather than smoothness, is used as a constraint (Brady & Yuille, 1983):[5]

$$E(X) = ||Y - X||^2 + \lambda(P^2/A). \tag{C.23}$$

In equation (C.23), A is a surface area enclosed by X and P is a total length (perimeter) of X. Minimizing P^2/A (or maximizing A/P^2) represents the classical isoperimetric problem (Polya & Szego, 1951). From all closed curves, a circle has a maximal area for a given perimeter or, conversely, has a minimal perimeter for a given area. Compactness involves the square of a perimeter, so that the ratio is not affected by changing the overall size of a figure. To illustrate the relation between 2D shape and its compactness, figure C.12 shows several planar figures along with the value of the compactness (A/P^2).

C.13   Bayesian Formulation of a Regularization Problem

If the visual noise on the retina is represented by a likelihood function $p(Y|X)$, and a priori knowledge of the family of possible solutions is repre-

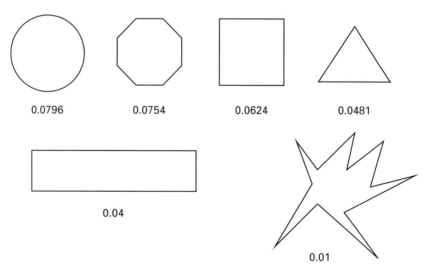

Figure C.12
Circularity index for several different figures with various degrees of regularity.

sented by probability distribution $p(X)$, then the visual data and a priori constraints can be combined by means of Bayes' rule (Knill & Richards, 1996):

$$p(X|Y) = p(Y|X)p(X)/p(Y). \tag{C.24}$$

Visual reconstruction of an object X can be obtained by finding X that maximizes $p(X|Y)$ (such an X is called a "maximum a posteriori" estimate). The denominator on the right-hand side in equation (C.24) is a constant and can be ignored in finding the maximum. If we take a negative log of both sides of (C.24), and ignore the denominator, we obtain

$$-\log[p(X|Y)] = -\log[p(Y|X)] - \log[p(X)]. \tag{C.25}$$

Since a logarithmic function is monotonic, maximizing the posterior in (C.24) leads to the same solution as minimizing the left-hand-side in (C.25). Note that equation (C.25) has the same form as equations (C.22) and (C.23). This observation leads to a more general statement that regularization and Bayesian methods are mathematically equivalent (Poggio et al., 1985). This equivalence can most clearly be seen if a regularization problem is expressed in the language of information theory. If we know the probabilities in equation (C.25), then we can find (at least in principle) an optimal description language that leads to the shortest expected length of the description of reconstructed objects (Leclerc, 1989; Chater, 1996; Li & Vitanyi, 1997). If the logarithms in equation (C.25) have the base of 2, the left-hand side is the length of a description of a given object. In this formalism, called "minimum description length," the reconstructed object is the one that has the shortest (most economical) description in a given language. Clearly, probabilities are used here to define simplicity. It follows that the controversy between simplicity and likelihood principles may be more difficult to resolve than originally thought (Hatfield & Epstein, 1985; Chater, 1996).

C.14   Examples of Application of Regularization Theory to 2.5D Sketch

First, consider reconstruction of 3D surface from depth measurements. Assume that the visual system has measurements of depth at a finite number of points on a continuous surface $f(x,y)$. These measurements are represented by a function $d(x,y)$, and they could be produced by binocular disparity, motion parallax, or other depth cues. The task is to reconstruct the surface $f(x,y)$. There are infinitely many different surfaces that can approximate a set of points in 3D. In order to obtain a unique surface, smoothness of the surface is used as a regularizing constraint. The reconstructed surface f is the one that minimizes the following cost function (Poggio et al., 1985; Grimson, 1982):

$$\int [(f - d)^2 + \lambda(f_{xx}^2 + 2f_{xy}^2 + f_{yy}^2)]dxdy. \qquad (C.26)$$

In equation (C.26) the smooth surface is the one whose second partial derivatives are close to zero everywhere. The cost function (C.26) for the case of a surface in 3D resembles the cost function (C.22) for the case of a contour in 2D. In both cases, smoothness is a constraint and this constraint is spatially local. Recall that for contours in 2D, a global constraint was proposed in the form of compactness (equation C.23), which seems to lead to equally good (or even better) reconstructions. There is no reason why reconstructing surfaces and shapes in 3D should not use an analogous constraint, expressed as the ratio of volume squared to total surface area cubed: V^2/S^3 (one should use the volume squared and surface area cubed to make this ratio size invariant). This constraint is called "3D compactness," and its role in modeling human shape perception is discussed in some detail in chapter 5.

Next, consider the problem of reconstructing 3D surface from shading (Ikeuchi & Horn, 1981). Assuming that the reflectance properties of the surface (e.g., that the surface is Lambertian) are known at least approximately, and that the position of the light source is known, Ikeuchi and Horn showed how the 2.5D sketch for a surface can be computed by using smoothness constraint. In this application, the 2.5D sketch is represented by surface orientations relative to the viewer. Surface orientation for a number of points in the image is computed by comparing the brightness distribution $E(x,y)$ in the image to the predicted brightness $R(x,y)$, which is a function of the surface orientation $f(x,y)$ and $g(x,y)$ at each point, as well as the position of the light source. The functions f and g represent the surface normal in stereographic projection. The inverse problem of reconstructing f and g is solved by finding the minimum of the following cost function:

$$\int [(E(x, y) - R(f, g))^2 + \lambda(f_x^2 + f_y^2 + g_x^2 + g_y^2)]dxdy. \qquad (C.27)$$

The smoothness constraint is expressed in equation (C.27) by the integral of squared derivatives of the surface gradients.

Finally, consider the reconstruction of the 2.5D sketch from binocular disparity. In this case, the 2.5D sketch corresponds to the function $d(x,y)$, which represents a continuous distribution of binocular disparity over a smooth surface. Let $L(x,y)$ and $R(x,y)$ be the brightness distribution on the left and right retina, correspondingly. When the vergence angle is close to zero, and there is no noise in the visual signal, $L(x,y) = R(x + d(x,y),y)$. This means that the corresponding points in the two retinas are shifted horizontally by d. To partially eliminate the effect of noise, which is always present in real images, the two retinal images are convolved with a Gaussian filter G. To emphasize the role of contours in the reconstruction, Laplacians of the brightness distributions are compared, rather than the brightness distributions themselves. The smoothness of the surface is represented by the requirement that the gradient of disparity be close to zero everywhere. The function $d(x,y)$ is reconstructed as a minimum of the following cost function (Poggio et al., 1985):

$$\int \{[\nabla^2 G*(L(x, y) - R(x + d(x, y), y), y))]^2 + \lambda(\nabla d)^2\}dxdy. \tag{C.28}$$

These three examples nicely illustrate the application of regularization methods in solving inverse problems of reconstructing 3D surfaces.

Appendix D: Shape Constraints in Reconstruction of Polyhedra

D.1   Chan, Stevenson, Li, and Pizlo's (2006) Model

The main part of the model is a reconstruction of a 3D shape H based on one retinal image I (see figure D.1 for a schematic illustration of the viewing geometry). A single 2D image determines infinitely many possible 3D shapes. In order to choose one, several constraints are used. The new model is an extension of Leclerc and Fischler's (1992) algorithm. In their algorithm, the 3D shape of a polyhedron was obtained from a single ortho-graphic image by taking the individual points of the 2D image and "moving" them along the lines orthogonal to the image plane. As a result, any 3D object produced by this algorithm is consistent with the given image under orthographic projection. From the infinite set of such objects, the algorithm chose the one that minimized some complexity measure represented by a cost function. This function had two components: the magnitude of the overall departure of reconstructed faces from planarity and the variance of all interior angles.

In the new model, a perspective rather than orthographic projection was used (a calibrated camera was assumed). The cost function included also the magnitude of the departure of the reconstructed object from a mirror symmetry. The cost function had the following form:

$$E_{mono}(H) = \gamma[VA(H) + DS(H)] + (1 - \gamma)DP(H), \tag{D.1}$$

where $VA(H)$ is the variance of all interior angles, $DP(H)$ is a measure of departure from planarity for all faces of H, $DS(H)$ is a measure of departure from mirror symmetry of H, and γ is a scalar that ranges from 0 to 1.

It is assumed in the model that the plane of symmetry is known. More exactly, it is assumed that it is known which angles are the symmetrical

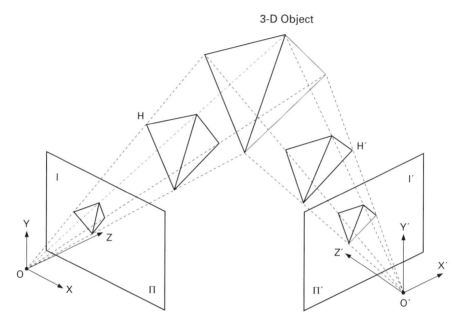

Figure D.1

A schematic diagram of Chan et al.'s shape reconstruction algorithm (from Pizlo, Li & Chan, 2005).

ones. The departure from mirror symmetry is computed as the sum of the squared differences between the corresponding angles over all pairs of angles in the polyhedron. The departure from planarity was measured by using a property of polygons, according to which the sum of all interior angles in an n-gon is equal to $(n - 2) \cdot 180$ deg. When a convex polygon is not planar, the sum of interior angles is smaller. Thus, the following expression is a measure of the departure from planarity of a convex n-gon (Leclerc & Fischler, 1992):

$$DP = \left[(n-2) \cdot 180 - \sum_j \alpha_j \right]^2. \qquad (D.2)$$

In equation (D.1), the term $DP(H)$ is the sum of the departure from planarity over all contours. Note that all three constraints are commensurate, that is, all use $(\deg)^2$ as a unit. The role of $DS(H)$ and $DP(H)$ in equation (D.1) is self-explanatory. The role of the variance of angles is less obvious. This term can be interpreted as a weak measure of symmetry of a polyhedron. This term was used for the first time by Marill (1991). He showed that minimum variance of angles by itself led to good reconstructions.

Leclerc and Fischler (1992) pointed out that this term is important in producing a volume of the reconstructed object. They added planarity constraint to improve the reconstructions.

Following Leclerc and Fischler (1992), a continuation method was used (Witkin et al., 1987; Leclerc, 1989) to minimize $E_{mono}(H)$. This method involves a sequence of descent steps applied to $E_{mono}(H)$ in which γ is decreased in each step. The algorithm starts with $\gamma \approx 1$. This means that the first step is strongly influenced by the $VA(H)$ and $DS(H)$ terms, which give the initial shape (volume) of H. As γ decreases, $DP(H)$ becomes the dominant factor, which enforces planarity of the faces. It is not desirable to emphasize planarity in the beginning of the reconstruction process. Note that the image itself is planar and thus represents a local minimum of the cost function (D.1). To "escape" from this minimum, planarity constraint is assigned a small weight in the beginning of the reconstruction. Note that planarity was used as an explicit constraint in the cost function. This was done so that the model could be applied to all polyhedral stimuli from the shape constancy experiments of Pizlo and his colleagues. Recall that some polyhedra had all contours planar, while others did not. Because each polyhedron had sixteen vertices, shape reconstruction involved fifteen independent parameters (sixteen points minus one). If planarity were used as an assumption, there would have been only three independent parameters.

In order to evaluate the role of the second image I', the model applied a correction to the reconstructed 3D shape H. This was done by projecting H to the plane of the second image and evaluating dissimilarity between this projected image and I'. The dissimilarity $SHI(I',H)$ involves the sum of squared differences between the angles of I' and the corresponding angles of H projected on the second camera image (see Chan et al., 2006, for details). The following cost function was used:

$$E_{bino}(H) = SHI(I',H) + \lambda[VA(H) + DS(H)]. \tag{D.3}$$

The model was tested with randomly generated polyhedra whose examples are shown in figure 4.9a and 4.9d–f. The model was not tested with stimuli (b) and (c) because in the case of these stimuli shape constraints cannot be applied. For example, the symmetry and planarity constraints cannot be applied to the polygonal line stimulus, and the application of the minimum variance of angles does not lead to a unique solution (see section D.2). Reconstructions of this model were compared to the reconstructions produced by an algorithm that reconstructs a 3D shape from binocular disparity, only, without any constraints.

There were three main results. First, monocular reconstructions of the new model were substantially better than binocular reconstructions of an algorithm that does not use any constraints. This result shows that shape constraints are more important in shape reconstruction than binocular disparity. Second, reliability of monocular reconstructions of the new model was correlated with human monocular and binocular performance. Specifically, the model's reconstructions were best for stimuli illustrated in figure 4.9a, second best for (e), then for (d) and worst for (f). Finally, reliability of binocular reconstructions of the new model did not correlate with human performance.

D.2 3D Shape Ambiguity When Constraints Are Used

What are the circumstances in which shape constraints may fail to produce a unique 3D shape? The issue of a uniqueness of perceptual interpretation was discussed in chapters 1 and 4 under the label of "shape ambiguity." When ellipses or triangles are used in a shape constancy experiment, the differences among the shapes within each of the two families are "not visible" from the point of view of the retinal image. As a result, the observer cannot discriminate among the shapes if only one 2D image is available. More generally, if the only difference among the stimuli is the depth of the stimulus, a single 2D image is not sufficient to discriminate among the stimuli. When more than one image is available, as in the case of a binocular observer, discrimination is possible in principle but is very unreliable in practice. How does this concept of shape ambiguity generalize to the case of shape reconstruction with the use of constraints? The main purpose of using constraints is to remove ambiguity related to depth. However, there is no constraint that can guarantee unambiguous interpretation with an arbitrary stimulus.

Consider the minimum-variance-of-angles constraint that was used in several studies, including that of Chan et al. (2006) (see the previous section). In the case of polyhedra, the minimum variance of angles leads to a unique solution (or at least to a finite number of solutions).[1] This is related to the fact that one cannot change the shape or 3D orientation of one face of a polyhedron without changing the shapes or orientations of other faces. The faces overconstrain one another. In other words, the shapes of the faces provide redundant information about the shape of the polyhedron. However, in the case of polygonal lines, such redundancy is absent. One can change one angle in the polygonal line without changing other angles. As a result, the minimum variance of angles leads to infinitely many solutions and, therefore, is not effective as a tool in solving an ill-posed inverse problem. Shape ambiguity arises and precludes studying shape constancy, the same way as using ellipses by Thouless and using elliptical cylinders by Johnston (1991) precluded them from studying shape constancy.

In the case of objects with smooth surfaces, variance of angles cannot be computed. But other shape properties can, like compactness (recall that compactness is defined as V^2/S^3, where V is the volume and S the surface area of the object). Consider the amoeba objects used by Edelman and Bülthoff (1992). The amoeba object is a sphere with a number of "spikes" around the surface of the sphere. Clearly, shifting one spike along the surface has no effect on the positions or sizes of other spikes. This is analogous to changing one angle in the polygonal line object without affecting angles in other parts of a polygonal line. At the same time, changing the position of one spike will not change such global shape measures as compactness: The total volume stays the same, as does the total surface area. It follows that the amoeba objects are also likely to lead to shape ambiguity.

In order to study shape constancy unconfounded with shape ambiguity, one has to understand not only the geometry of perspective projection but also the nature of shape constraints that are used by the visual system. The problem is, however, that we do not really know what these constraints are. This may explain, at least partially, why the progress in studying shape perception was slow: *In order to design the right experiment on shape, one has to know the nature of shape constraints one is trying to discover in that experiment!* Some of the most influential students of vision recognized this problem. For example, Brunswik (1956) and Gibson (1979) strongly emphasized the ecological validity of experimental stimuli. It is quite possible that objects in our natural environment never lead to shape ambiguity. If this were true, it would explain why shape constancy is the rule in our everyday life, and failures of shape constancy, including shape illusions, are exceedingly rare.

Notes

Chapter 1

1. This is a commonly accepted definition of "shape constancy." The reader can find it in textbooks of perception (e.g., Palmer, 1999; Levine, 2000; Schiffman, 2001) and in books on perceptual constancy (Epstein, 1977; Walsh & Kulikowski, 1998), as well as in classical sources such as Koffka (1935), Gibson (1950), Arnheim (1969), Zusne (1970), or Pastore (1971).

2. It seems unlikely that all of these ideas and observations were first made by Alhazen. Many, perhaps even most, may have been common knowledge among physicians before Alhazen passed them down in his book that survived the late Middle Ages.

3. Boring (1929, 1950) and others preferred the term "unconscious inference" or even "unconscious reasoning" (rather than "unconscious conclusion") as his preferred translation of *unbewusster Schluss*. The dictionary translation of *Schluss* is as an "end" or "conclusion." Conversely, "conclusion" is translated as *Schluss*. "Inference" seems to be a permissible translation of *Schluss*, but it does not seem to be as good as "conclusion." "Reasoning" does not seem right at all. My preference is to use "conclusion." Obviously, it does not really matter which expression we use, as long as we know the nature of the mechanisms Helmholtz' used in his theory. It is worthwhile, however, to keep in mind that such terms as "inference," "reasoning," "mental representation," and "information processing" were introduced into psychological models of perceptual processes after the Cognitive Revolution (Bruner et al., 1956; Miller et al., 1960; Epstein, 1973; Marr, 1982; Rock, 1983). With this in mind, it is clear that the theory presented in the paragraph quoted refers to something like Pavlovian conditioning, or Hebbian learning, more than reasoning or inference.

4. The same would be true if triangles were used. The shape of triangles is characterized by two parameters, and they lead to exactly the same problems as ellipses, whose shape is characterized by one parameter.

5. In Experiment 3, Stavrianos used smaller rectangles. By doing this, she effectively introduced shape ambiguity because small rectangles are approximately equivalent under perspective projection. It follows that her Experiment 3 did not study shape constancy but rather shape ambiguity.

6. These results indicate that subjects can, in fact, consciously judge the magnitude of slant. This conflicts with unconscious conclusion or inference theories in which slant (or experience related to it) is unconsciously taken into account in perception of shape, as claimed by Helmholtz (1867/2000) and Rock (1983). If the subjects did not have conscious access to the information about slant, slant judgments would be equally poor across the reduction conditions. These judgments, however, were more precise and accurate in the presence of depth cues than in their absence as one would expect.

7. Note that this conjecture runs in exactly the opposite direction to that of the traditional view of "taking into account," according to which slant is taken into account in determining the perceived shape. Stavrianos' point is that shape could be taken into account in determining the perceived slant.

8. This conjecture, which was "picked-up" by Gibson, provided him with stimulation throughout his entire career (Gibson, 1950, 1966, 1979).

9. Comparison of shape ambiguity to shape constancy with planar figures has been replicated more recently by the present author, confirming all claims derived from Thouless' and Stavrianos' experiments (Pizlo, 1994; Pizlo & Salach-Golyska, 1995; Pizlo & Scheessele, 1998).

10. The constancy hypothesis is completely unrelated to the phenomenon called "perceptual constancy."

11. See Steinman, Pizlo, and Pizlo (2000) for a recent presentation and discussion of Wertheimer's 1912 contribution.

12. It is worth pointing out that sometimes the path of light maximizes time. Therefore, it is better to talk about the principle of stationary, rather than minimum, time.

13. In chapter 3 it will be shown, however, how the "minimum principle," when used as a constraint within a regularization theory, can be used to formulate modern computational models of perceptual mechanisms. In particular, Poggio et al. (1985) showed that at least some perceptual mechanisms can be modeled by electrical circuits, where the percept is "explained" by the state of the circuit corresponding to the minimum amount of heat generated in resistors.

14. This experiment was replicated by Hochberg and McAlister (1953). They used better methodology, and their results were put in the framework of information theory (see chapter 2).

Chapter 2

1. Tolman would have been offended by having his name listed along with Hugo Münsterberg's because he considered Münsterberg's writings about purposive behavior to be unscientific. It is worth pointing out, however, that Münsterberg's understanding of the relation between determinism and purposive actions (see his chapter 21, pp. 285–296) was very close to the modern treatment of this relation as held by Wiener and his colleagues (Rosenblueth, Wiener, & Bigelow, 1943).

2. First, note that figure 2.1a is not exactly consistent with a cube interpretation. Instead, it is consistent with a rectangular box, whose faces are not all identical. Second, note that there are infinitely many 2D and 3D interpretations corresponding to each drawing. The set of these interpretations contains planar figures with various slants and tilts as well as polyhedral and nonpolyhedral objects. In fact, a given 2D image can be produced by a set of unrelated points in three dimensions, rather than a set of lines or quadrilaterals. It so happens that when a 2D image on the retina can be produced by a cube, the observer perceives a cube, rather than any of the other 2D or 3D possible interpretations. Hochberg and McAlister did not discuss the simplicity rule (criterion) responsible for this perceptual choice. The first formulation of such a rule was put forth by Perkins (1972, 1976) and was subsequently elaborated by Sinha and Adelson (1992), Leclerc and Fischler (1992), and Marill (1991). The most recent version was provided by Pizlo, Li, and Chan (2005), Chan et al. (2006), and Li and Pizlo (2006).

3. Hochberg and McAlister, in their table 1, reported the number of angles minus one, rather than the number of angles itself. Also note a typo in this table. For figure (c), their table indicates, incorrectly, 17 junction points. This typo was corrected in the later reprint of this paper in Beardslee and Wertheimer (1958).

4. Koffka's (1935) ideas about the conflict of internal and external forces in perception apparently influenced Attneave and Frost's thinking. Later, it will be shown that the percept is not a result of conflict between the retinal image and simplicity. Instead, simplicity is needed to obtain a veridical, 3D percept from a 2D retinal image.

5. Note that the Y junction in figure 2.6 may be perceived as a right trihedral angle, and indeed, the junction itself could be a projection of such an angle.

6. In the case of an orthographic projection, when a solution exists, there is a complementary solution corresponding to a depth reversal.

7. Interestingly, it was just such unstructured objects that Rock and DiVita (1987) and Edelman and Bülthoff (1992) used for studies in which they demonstrated a failure of shape constancy. Note that their decision to use unstructured wire objects to study shape constancy was analogous to the use of ellipses and triangles by Thouless (1931a, b) in his studies.

8. Hebb's motor theory of shape perception was subsequently elaborated by Festinger (Festinger et al., 1967; Festinger, 1971; but see also Miller & Festinger, 1977) and by Stark (e.g., Noton & Stark, 1971). All modern motor theories are very closely related to Lotze's (1852) theory of local signs, in which he tried to explain the ability of the visual system to judge relative positions on the retina, and to Helmholtz' (1867/2000) elaboration of Lotze's theory to the case of orientation and curvature of retinal lines. Motor theories of shape perception have never been applied to 3D shapes, nor is it clear that they could be. For this reason, this line of research was left out of this book.

9. Gregory (1970, 1980) held a similar position to that of Rock. Gregory viewed the visual system as a "scientist" who is solving problems by formulating hypotheses and testing them. Testing perceptual hypotheses might involve interaction with the environment. In this way, Gregory's theory made a provision for the role of experience in visual perception.

Chapter 3

1. Machine vision (also called "robot" or "computer" vision) is relevant for understanding human vision and vice versa. Both communities, made up primarily of engineers and psychologists, respectively, are trying to develop a theory of visual perception. Psychologists are seeking a theory of biological (human) vision, whereas engineers are seeking a theory of artificial vision. Despite the obvious similarity of the overall goal of both lines of research, interaction between these two communities has never been strong. The main reason seems to derive from the very different methodology used in human and machine vision research. Psychologists and engineers go about their work quite differently; engineers do simulations, while psychologists perform psychophysical experiments. The main differences between these very different approaches to vision, as well as their strengths and limitations, are tabulated in appendix C.1a (after Pizlo, Rosenfeld, & Weiss, 1995).

2. Roberts credits Gibson (1950) for inspiring his work—in particular, for shifting attention from 2D figures to 3D objects and for suggesting that projective geometry might be useful for addressing the issue of shape constancy.

3. Homogeneous coordinates allow one to handle the numerators and the denominator separately in a perspective projection. In particular, since all equations in a perspective projection involve the same denominator, a "spurious" dimension is introduced that represents this denominator. The remaining dimensions represent the numerators. As a result, a perspective projection from a 3D scene to the 2D image can be represented by a set of linear equations, in which the 3D Euclidean coordinates describing the objects "out there" are replaced by 4D homogeneous coordinates, and similarly, the 2D Euclidean coordinates on the retina are replaced by 3D homogeneous coordinates.

4. This corresponds to the distinction between a calibrated and an uncalibrated camera. In a calibrated camera, the geometry of the camera, including the focal distance, is known, and as a result, Euclidean structure can be recognized (Pizlo & Loubier, 2000). In an uncalibrated camera, the geometry of the camera is not known, and as a result, Euclidean structure is not accessible. The case of an uncalibrated camera received a lot of attention in the computer vision community (e.g., Faugeras, 1993), but it has no application in human vision—see appendix C, section C.4.

5. This similarity is related to the fact that colinearity and coplanarity, the features used explicitly in the reconstruction methods of Waltz and others, are actually projective invariants. It follows that when a polyhedron is reconstructed from a single image, the reconstruction *often* leads to a family of polyhedra that are projectively equivalent. Specifically, the family of reconstructed polyhedra is larger than the family of projectively equivalent shapes when the polyhedron has a complex shape (e.g., when there are vertices produced by four or more faces). However, for simple polyhedra, such as hexahedrons, or for parts of a complex polyhedron, the family of reconstructed polyhedra consists of objects that are projectively equivalent. This is related to the fact that for simple polyhedra, planarity of faces is the only constraint that defines 3D projective transformations. This can be illustrated in the case of a hexahedron with quadrilateral faces (such as a cube or parallelepiped), where planarity of faces (including coplanarity of quadruples of points on diagonals) is the only constraint that generates the family of projectively equivalent objects (M. Brill, personal communication). The relation between reconstruction of a 3D shape from a single image and a group of 3D projective transformations provided the basis for formulating model-based projective invariants for 3D shapes and will be discussed in some more detail in section 3.3).

6. Problems with using Marr's 2.5D sketch as the basis for shape perception arise not only when edges are used but also when surfaces are used, although it is not as easy to provide compelling illustrations. It is known that perceived 3D slants of planar surfaces are systematically underestimated (see Perrone, 1980, 1982, for a review). If the perceived shape of an object were derived from the percept of the object's surfaces, one would expect systematic errors in judging 3D shapes of objects. Look at figure 2.4. When the 3D orientation of the planes π_1, π_2, and π_3 are underestimated, the trihedral angle formed by these planes should not be perceived as a right angle. But it is. Specifically, Perkins showed no systematic errors either in perception of right trihedral angles (1972) or in perception of arbitrary angles of regular polyhedra (1976). Perceived shape of a polyhedron is more accurate than perceived orientations of surfaces and edges (see chapter 4, where a direct psychophysical test is described). It follows that 3D shape is not derived from 2.5D representation. In perception of 3D shapes, regularity of the shape is more important than information about depth and 3D orientation of surfaces and edges.

7. When the cameras are uncalibrated, the 3D projective, but not Euclidean, structure can be computed (Hartley & Zisserman, 2003).

8. A unique solution requires only six points. When seven or more points are available, the computations are easier than in the case of six points (Tsai & Huang, 1984).

9. The fact that shape is not affected by rigid motion is an example of von Ehrenfels' transposition principle (see chapter 1). It follows that mathematical (conventional) invariants provide an explanation of the transposition principle. Note, however, that shape constancy does not simply follow from the transposition principle, a fact overlooked by almost everyone, including Gibson (1966), Boring (1942), and Zusne (1970).

10. This statement applies only to the perception of 3D shape from a single 2D image. If two or more 2D images are available, 3D projective invariants can be computed (Faugeras, 1993). In other words, a transformation from a 3D space to two camera images, when the cameras are uncalibrated, can be treated as a 3D projectivity. When two calibrated cameras are used, this transformation can be treated as a similarity transformation of a 3D space (Longuet-Higgins, 1981).

11. It seems likely that the problems that arise when projective invariants are used to explain shape constancy did not become obvious until recently because of the persistent prevalence of "taking slant into account" explanations (see chapter 1).

12. Despite some initial enthusiasm (for a review, see Mundy & Zisserman, 1992; Mundy et al., 1993), it became obvious that projective invariants have fundamental limitations not only as an explanation of human shape perception but also as a tool in engineering applications (see appendix C, section C.6, for a review of the use of projective invariants in machine vision).

13. When the range in depth of a slanted figure is small as compared to the viewing distance, perspective projection can be approximated by a 2D affine transformation. In such a case, affine invariants can be used as an approximation of perspective invariants. The relevance of affine invariants under such conditions was demonstrated by Wagemans et al. (2000).

14. Pizlo and Loubier (2000) were able to formulate a 3D perspective model-based invariant (appendix C, section C.9.2, provides a brief treatment). This perspective invariant does not suffer from this problem. However, it can only be applied to one object at a time, instead of to the entire class of objects. Specifically, this invariant provides an answer to the question of whether a given perspective image was produced by a given 3D object. The potential value of using this 3D perspective invariant for the study of human shape constancy has not been tested yet.

15. Hume (1739) was probably the first philosopher to have realized the nature of this problem. He insisted that the causality relation in physics cannot be *perceptually* observed. It can only be postulated (*inferred*), but empirical data will never be able to prove a causal relation in natural phenomena. A standard way to alleviate Hume's

problem is to use a simplicity principle (Occam's razor). The framework of inverse problems in visual perception, the Prägnanz principle of Gestalt psychologists, and the Occam's razor principle in natural sciences are different names for the same solution of the problem posed by Hume.

16. This property of a circle is represented by an isoperimetric inequality (Polya & Szego, 1951).

Chapter 4

1. The fact that binocular disparity is used across objects (i.e., across spatial discontinuities), but not within objects, invalidates theories of binocular visual space, such as Luneburg's (1947). In Luneburg's theory there is one global geometrical model describing perceived 3D spatial relations regardless of the stimuli and the task. In his theory, the same perceptual distortions must be observed across objects as within them.

2. Marr (1977) proposed the following four characteristics to describe generalized cones: (i) shape of a cross section, (ii) shape of the axis, (iii) axial scaling function, and (iv) eccentricity angle. For example, the circular cylinder (figure 4.7c) has a circular cross section, its axis is straight, the size of its cross section is constant, and the cross section of this shape is orthogonal to its axis. A circular cone (figure 4.7a) is different from a circular cylinder in that the size of the cross section is not constant. Realize that Marr's definition of generalized cones can be generalized even further. For example, the cross section may vary not only with respect to its size but also with respect to shape. Furthermore, the eccentricity angle does not have to be kept constant. With such generalizations, however, the family of generalized cones becomes very large—so large that it is not clear that it can be used in machine (or human) shape recognition systems (see, e.g., Koenderink, 1995, for a criticism of limitations inherent in the concept of generalized cones).

3. Watt (1987) showed that the Weber fraction in line-length discrimination, when the lines are presented in a frontal plane, is about 10% when exposure duration is 100 ms. In order to achieve very reliable discrimination in the line-length experiment (Weber fraction of 2%–3%), exposure duration has to be about 1 second or more.

4. The effect of experimental conditions on performance was the same when overall proportion of correct responses was used as a dependent variable.

Chapter 5

1. D'Arcy Thompson (1942) remarked, "symmetry is highly characteristic of organic forms, and is rarely absent in living things—save in such few cases as Amoeba" (p. 357).

2. This argument is analogous to the one presented by Bennett, Hoffman, and Prakash (1989, 1991) in their "observer mechanics" theory. The main difference is that they used constraints in the form of assumptions, like the rigidity assumption in Ullman's (1979) theory. Here, constraints are used explicitly as an element of a regularization model.

3. It was shown in appendix C.11 that when a planarity constraint is applied to an image of a simple polyhedron, there are only three degrees of freedom characterizing the 3D shape of this polyhedron. The same is true with shapes like geons that were used by Biederman (1985), as well as with other generalized cones and superquadrics. Examples of computational methods that illustrate how simple generalized cones and superquadrics are reconstructed can be found in Chakravarty (1979), Malik and Maydan (1989), Dickinson and Metaxas (1994), Ulupinar and Nevatia (1995), and Zerroug and Nevatia (1996, 1999).

4. This statement actually applies to an orthographic projection. A perspective image of a symmetrical object uniquely determines the object. However, in the presence of visual noise, a reconstruction is likely to be unstable. Thus, additional constraints are needed for reconstruction when either projection is used.

5. It seems likely that with natural objects, planarity is subordinate to symmetry. Objects and structures that have planar contours but no symmetry are not common in nature. Even artificial objects are almost always symmetric, simply because mechanical stability, in the presence of gravity, requires symmetry.

6. Quite a lot is known in geometry about compactness. It was studied quite extensively as an element of isoperimetric inequalities (Polya & Szego, 1951). Isoperimetric inequalities analysis is a treatment of geometrical and physical properties of objects, such as their shapes, symmetries, and rigidity. This kind of analysis has established that symmetry and convexity of an object, as well as smoothness of its surface, lead to greater compactness.

7. The only prior application of compactness in shape reconstruction was the use of a 2D compactness constraint that was applied to a slanted circle (Brady & Yuille, 1983), or to other slanted figures that were cross sections of generalized cylinders (Dickinson & Metaxas, 1994; Ulupinar & Nevatia, 1995), described in chapter 3. Sinha (1995) also used the term "compactness" when he presented his new constraint. However, his "compactness" constraint was completely different from the constraint used in this book. He used a constraint that biased the faces of polyhedra towards small slants, relative to the camera. This constraint would be more appropriately called a "depth constraint," not a compactness constraint. The use of the term "compactness" in this book is completely different. It is novel because it refers to *3D* compactness.

8. There are, actually, two objects in which the angles are all 90 deg angles. One is a box viewed from outside, and the other is a box viewed from inside (convex vs.

concave). Note that only one of these two interpretations is seen by the observer. The visual system uses an assumption (constraint) that objects are always seen from outside (Mamassian & Landy, 1998).

9. The examples presented here use an orthographic projection as an approximation to a perspective projection. This approximation, however, does not restrict the generality of these examples.

10. In this example, departure from symmetry, DS, was measured by the mean squared difference between the angles of the object and the 90 deg angle (the angles were expressed in degrees). The cost function was as follows: $E = DS - V^2/S^3$.

11. When a perspective image of a bilaterally symmetrical object is given, the object can, in principle, be reconstructed uniquely by applying Longuet-Higgins' (1981) algorithm (see chapter 3). However, such a reconstruction will be unstable, so it cannot be veridical. One has to use additional constraints, such as compactness, to stabilize the result from this kind of reconstruction.

Appendix C

1. It is assumed here, for simplicity, that the surface of the retina is planar, even though it is actually spherical. This assumption does not restrict the generality of the derivation because one can always transform mathematically a spherical image to a planar one, and vice versa.

2. If you get too close, you will not be able to accommodate and the shape will be blurred. To overcome the accommodation problem, the reader can project a copy of this image on a large screen and look at it from a distance at which the image occupies a large part of the visual field.

3. In order to make statements about the probability of events, one would have to make assumptions about the probability distributions over objects and viewing orientations. In our case, however, fairly weak assumptions would be needed such as that most viewing orientations are observed with a probability greater than zero.

4. Interestingly, the method for objects with bilateral symmetry cannot be applied to solids of revolution. When the line of sight intersects the axis of symmetry of a solid of revolution, the two symmetrical halves of the image are, by definition, identical, except for mirror symmetry. Therefore, they are completely redundant and cannot be used to perform a reconstruction from two views. As pointed out earlier, any other perspective image of a solid of revolution is a 2D projective transformation of the symmetrical image, and therefore the redundancy problem applies to it, as well.

5. Brady and Yuille (1983) used this constraint in the context of reconstructing slanted figures, rather than interpolating retinal images, as described here. The same

constraint was used by Ulupinar and Nevatia (1995) and Dickinson and Metaxas (1994) in reconstructing generalized cones.

Appendix D

1. Usually, there are two solutions corresponding to the depth reversal. In the general case, however, it is difficult to establish the number of minima of the variance of angles in a polyhedron. Based on computational experiments, it seems that in the case of simple polyhedra, there are only two minima.

References

Alhazen (1083/1989) *The optics of Ibm Al-Haytham: Books 1–3*. (Translated by A. I. Sabra.) London: Warburg Institute.

Alter, T. D. & Basri, R. (1998) Extracting salient curves from images: An analysis of the saliency network. *International Journal of Computer Vision*, 27, 51–69.

Arnheim, R. (1969) *Visual thinking*. Berkeley: University of California Press.

Ashby, W. R. (1940) Adaptiveness and equilibrium. *Journal of Mental Science*, 86, 478–483.

Astrom, K. (1995) Fundamental limitations on projective invariants of planar curves. *IEEE Transactions on Pattern Analysis and Machine Intelligence*, 17, 77–81.

Attneave, F. (1954) Some informational aspects of visual perception. *Psychological Review*, 61, 183–193.

Attneave, F. (1959) *Applications of information theory to psychology*. New York: Holt.

Attneave, F. & Frost, R. (1969) The determination of perceived tridimensional orientation by minimum criteria. *Perception & Psychophysics*, 6, 391–396.

Backus, B. T., Banks, M. S., van Ee, R. & Crowell, J. A. (1999) Horizontal and vertical disparity, eye position, and stereoscopic slant perception. *Vision Research*, 39, 1143–1170.

Ballard, D. H. & Brown, C. M. (1982) *Computer vision*. Englewood Cliffs, NJ: Prentice Hall.

Barlow, H. B. (1961) Possible principles underlying the transformations of sensory messages. In: Rosenblith, W. A. (Ed.) *Sensory communication* (pp. 217–234). New York: Wiley.

Barrow, H. G. & Tenenbaum, J. M. (1981) Interpreting line drawings as three-dimensional surfaces. *Artificial Intelligence*, 17, 75–116.

Basri, R. & Ullman, S. (1993) The alignment of objects with smooth surfaces. *CVGIP: Image Understanding*, 57, 331–345.

Beardslee, D. C. & Wertheimer, M. (1958) *Readings in perception*. New York: D. van Nostrand.

Beck, J. & Gibson, J. J. (1955) The relation of apparent shape to apparent slant in the perception of objects. *Journal of Experimental Psychology*, 50, 125–133.

Bennett, B. M., Hoffman, D. D. & Prakash, C. (1989) *Observer mechanics*. New York: Academic Press.

Bennett, B. M., Hoffman, D. D. & Prakash, C. (1991) Unity of perception. *Cognition*, 38, 295–334.

Bennett, S. (1979) *A history of control engineering 1800–1930*. London: Peregrinus.

Bennett, S. (1993) *A history of control engineering 1930–1955*. Stevenage: Peregrinus.

Bergevin, R. & Levine, M. D. (1992a) Part decomposition of objects from single view line drawings. *CVGIP: Image Understanding*, 55, 73–83.

Bergevin, R. & Levine, M. D. (1992b) Extraction of line drawing features for object recognition. *Pattern Recognition*, 25, 319–334.

Bergevin, R. & Levine, M. D. (1993) Generic object recognition: Building and matching coarse 3D descriptions from line drawings. *IEEE Transactions on Pattern Analysis and Machine Intelligence*, 15, 19–36.

Berkeley, G. (1709/1910) *A new theory of vision*. New York: Dutton.

Biederman, I. (1985) Human image understanding: Recent research and a theory. *Computer Vision, Graphics, and Image Processing*, 32, 29–73.

Biederman, I. (1987) Recognition-by-components: A theory of human image understanding. *Psychological Review*, 94, 115–147.

Biederman, I. & Gerhardstein, P. C. (1993) Recognizing depth-rotated objects: Evidence and conditions from three-dimensional viewpoint invariance. *Journal of Experimental Psychology: Human Perception and Performance*, 19, 1162–1182.

Binford, T. O. (1971) Visual perception by computer. *IEEE Conference on Systems and Control*. Miami.

Blum, H. (1973) Biological shape and visual science. *Journal of Theoretical Biology*, 38, 205–287.

Borges, D. L. & Fisher, R. B. (1997) Class-based recognition of 3d objects represented by volumetric primitives. *Image Vision Computing*, 15, 655–664.

Boring, E. G. (1929) *A history of experimental psychology*, first edition. New York: Appleton.

Boring, E. G. (1942) *Sensation and perception in the history of experimental psychology*. New York: Appleton.

Boring, E. G. (1950) *A history of experimental psychology*, second edition. New York: Appleton.

Boyer, K. L. & Sarkar, S. (1999) Perceptual organization in computer vision: Status, challenges, and potential. *Computer Vision & Image Understanding*, 76, No. 1.

Boyer, K. L. & Sarkar, S. (2000) *Perceptual organization for artificial vision systems*. Boston: Kluwer.

Bradshaw, M. F., Parton, A. D. & Glennerster, A. (2000) The task-dependent use of binocular disparity and motion parallax information. *Vision Research*, 40, 3725–3734.

Brady, J. M. (1981) *Computer vision*. Amsterdam: North Holland.

Brady, M. & Yuille, A. (1983) Inferring 3D orientation from 2D contour (an extremum principle). In: Richards, W. (Ed.) *Natural computation* (pp. 99–106). Cambridge: MIT Press.

Braithwaite, R. B. (1955) *Scientific explanation*. Cambridge: Cambridge University Press.

Braunstein, M. (1976) *Depth perception through motion*. New York: Academic Press.

Bribiesca, E. (2000) A measure of compactness for 3D shapes. *Computers & Mathematics with Applications*, 40, 1275–1284.

Bruner, J. S. (1957) Going beyond the information given. In: Gruber, H., Hammond, K. R. & Jesser, R. (Eds.) *Contemporary approaches to cognition*. Cambridge: Harvard University Press.

Bruner, J. S. & Goodman, C. C. (1947) Value and need as organizing factors in perception. *Journal of Abnormal and Social Psychology*, 42, 33–44.

Bruner, J. S., Goodnow, J. J. & Austin, G. A. (1956) *A study of thinking*. New York: Wiley.

Brunswik, E. (1944) Distal focusing of perception: Size-constancy in a representative sample of situations. *Psychological Monographs*, 56, No. 254.

Brunswik, E. (1956) *Perception and the representative design of psychological experiments*. Berkeley: University of California Press.

Bülthoff, H. H. (1991) Shape from X: Psychophysics and computation. In: Landy, M. S. & Movshon, J. A. (Eds.) *Computational models of visual processing* (pp. 305–330). Cambridge: MIT Press.

Bülthoff, H. H. & Edelman, S. (1992) Psychophysical support for a two-dimensional view interpolation theory of object recognition. *Proceedings of the National Academy of Sciences*, 89, 60–64.

Bülthoff, H. H. & Mallot, H. A. (1988) Integration of depth modules: Stereo and shading. *Journal of the Optical Society of America*, A5, 1749–1758.

Burns, J. B., Weiss, R. & Riseman, E. M. (1990) View variation of point set and line segment features. *Proceedings of DARPA Image Understanding Workshop*, 650–659.

Cannon, W. B. (1932) *The wisdom of the body*. New York: Norton.

Cantril, H. (1960) *The morning notes of Adelbert Ames, Jr.* New Brunswick, NJ: Rutgers University Press.

Cassirer, E. (1938/1944) The concept of group and the theory of perception. *Philosophy and Phenomenological Research*, 5, 1–35.

Chakravarty, I. (1979) A generalized line and junction labeling scheme with applications to scene analysis. *IEEE Transactions on Pattern Analysis and Machine Intelligence*, 1, 202–205.

Chakravarty, I. & Freeman, H. (1982) Characteristic views as a basis for three-dimensional object recognition. Proceedings, SPIE Conference on Robot Vision, pp. 37–45, Arlington VA.

Chan, M. W., Stevenson, A. K., Li, Y. & Pizlo, Z. (2006) Binocular shape constancy from novel views: The role of *a priori* constraints. *Perception & Psychophysics*, 68, 1124–1139.

Chater, N. (1996) Reconciling simplicity and likelihood principles in perceptual organization. *Psychological Review*, 103, 566–581.

Cherry, C. (1978) *On human communication*. Cambridge: MIT Press.

Clark, J. J. & Yuille, A. L. (1990) *Data fusion for sensory information processing systems*. Boston: Kluwer.

Clowes, M. B. (1971) On seeing things. *Artificial Intelligence*, 2, 79–116.

Courant, R. & Robbins, H. (1941) *What is mathematics?* New York: Oxford University Press.

Craik, K. J. W. (1943) *The nature of explanation*. Cambridge: Cambridge University Press.

Descartes, R. (1637/2001) *Discourse on method, optics, geometry, and meteorology*. (Translated by P. J. Olscamp.) Indianapolis: Hackett.

Dewey, J. (1896) The reflex arc concept in psychology. *Psychological Review*, 3, 357–370.

Dickinson, S., Bergevin, R., Biederman, I., Eklundh, J.-O., Jain, A., Munck-Fairwood, R. & Pentland, A. (1997) Panel report: The potential of geons for generic 3-D object recognition. *Image and Vision Computing*, 15, 277–292.

Dickinson, S. & Metaxas, D. (1994) Integrating qualitative and quantitative shape recovery. *International Journal of Computer Vision*, 13, 311–330.

Dickinson, S., Metaxas, D. & Pentland, A. (1997) The role of model-based segmentation in the recovery of volumetric parts from range data. *IEEE Transactions on Pattern Analysis and Machine Intelligence*, 19, 259–267.

Dickinson, S., Pentland, A. & Rosenfeld, A. (1990) A representation for qualitative 3-D object recognition integrating object-centered and viewer-centered models. In: Leibovic, K. (Ed.) *Vision: A convergence of disciplines* (pp. 398–421). New York: Springer-Verlag.

Dickinson, S., Pentland, A. & Rosenfeld, A. (1992a) 3-D shape recovery using distributed aspect matching. *IEEE Transactions on Pattern Analysis and Machine Intelligence*, 14, 174–198.

Dickinson, S., Pentland, A. & Rosenfeld, A. (1992b) From volumes to views: An approach to 3-D object recognition. *CVGIP: Image Understanding*, 55, 130–154.

Doorschot, P. C. A., Kappers, A. M. L. & Koenderink, J. J. (2001) The combined influence of binocular disparity and shading on pictorial shape. *Perception & Psychophysics*, 63, 1038–1047.

Du, L. & Munck-Fairwood, R. (1993) A formal definition and framework for generic object recognition. *Proceedings, 8th Scandinavian Conference on Image Analysis*, University of Tromsö, Norway.

Du, L. & Munck-Fairwood, R. (1995) Geon recognition through robust feature grouping. *Proceedings, 9th Scandinavian Conference on Image Analysis*, Uppsala, Sweden.

Duda, R. O. & Hart, P. E. (1973) *Pattern classification and scene analysis*. New York: Wiley.

Durgin, F. H., Proffitt, D. R., Olson, T. J. & Reinke, K. S. (1995) Comparing depth from motion with depth from binocular disparity. *Journal of Experimental Psychology: Human Perception and Performance*, 21, 679–699.

Edelman, S. & Bülthoff, H. H. (1992) Orientation dependence in the recognition of familiar and novel views of 3D objects. *Vision Research*, 32, 2385–2400.

Ee, R. van, van Dam, L. C. J. & Erkelens, C. J. (2002) Bi-stability in perceived slant when binocular disparity and monocular perspective specify different slants. *Journal of Vision*, 2, 597–607.

Eggert, D. & Bowyer, K. (1990) Computing the orthographic projection aspect graph of solids of revolution. *Pattern Recognition Letters*, 11, 751–763.

Eggert, D., Bowyer, K., Dyer, C., Christensen, H. & Goldgof, D. (1993) The scale space aspect graph. *IEEE Transactions on Pattern Analysis and Machine Intelligence*, 15, 1114–1130.

Ehrenfels, C. von (1890) Uber Gestaltqualitäten. *Vierteljahrschrift für Wissenschaftliche Philosophie*, 14, 249–292.

Eklundh, J.-O. & Olofsson, G. (1992) *Geon-based recognition in an active vision system.* ESPRIT-BRA 3038, Vision as Process. Springer-Verlag ESPRIT Series.

Epstein, W. (1973) The process of "taking-into-account" in visual perception. *Perception*, 2, 267–285.

Epstein, W. (1977) Stability and constancy in visual perception. New York: Wiley.

Epstein, W., Bontrager, H. & Park, J. (1962) The induction of nonveridical slant and the perception of shape. *Journal of Experimental Psychology*, 63, 472–479.

Farah, M. J., Rochlin, R. & Klein, K. L. (1994) Orientation invariance and geometric primitives in shape recognition. *Cognitive Science*, 18, 325–344.

Faugeras, O. (1993) *Three-dimensional computer vision.* Cambridge: MIT Press.

Fechner, G. (1860/1966) *Elements of psychophysics.* New York: Holt, Rinehart & Winston.

Feigenbaum, E. A. & Feldman, J. (1963) *Computers and thought.* New York: McGraw-Hill.

Festinger, L. (1971) Eye movements and perception. In: Bach-y-Rita, P. & Collins, C. C. (Eds.) *The control of eye movements* (pp. 259–273). New York: Academic Press.

Festinger, L., Burnham, C. A., Ono, H. & Bamber, D. (1967) Efference and the conscious experience of perception. *Journal of Experimental Psychology Monograph*, 3, 1–36.

Fitts, P. M. (1954) The information capacity of the human motor system in controlling the amplitude of movement. *Journal of Experimental Psychology*, 47, 281–391.

Gardner, H. (1987) *The mind's new science.* New York: Basic Books.

Gibson, J. J. (1950) *The perception of the visual world.* Boston: Houghton Mifflin.

Gibson, J. J. (1966) *The senses considered as perceptual systems.* Boston: Houghton Mifflin.

Gibson, J. J. (1979) *The ecological approach to visual perception.* Boston: Houghton Mifflin.

Ginsburg, A. P. (1986) Spatial filtering and visual form perception. In: Boff, K. R., Kaufman, L. & Thomas, J. P. (Eds.) *Handbook of perception and human performance* (chapter 34). New York: Wiley.

Glennerster, A., Rogers, B. J. & Bradhaw, M. F. (1996) Stereoscopic depth constancy depends on the subject's task. *Vision Research*, 36, 3441–3456.

Gottheil, E. & Bitterman, M. E. (1951) The measurement of shape-constancy. *American Journal of Psychology*, 64, 406–408.

Gregory, R. L. (1968) Visual illusions. *Scientific American*, 219, 66–76.

Gregory, R. L. (1970) *The intelligent eye*. New York: McGraw-Hill.

Gregory, R. L. (1980) Perceptions as hypotheses. *Philosophical Transactions of the Royal Society, London*, B290, 181–197.

Grimson, W. E. L. (1982) A computational theory of visual surface interpolation. *Philosophical Transactions of the Royal Society, London*, B298, 395–427.

Grossberg, S. & Mingolla, E. (1985) Neural dynamics of form perception: Boundary completion, illusory figures, and neon color spreading. *Psychological Review*, 92, 173–211.

Guy, G. & Medioni, G. (1996) Inferring global perceptual contours from local features. *International Journal of Computer Vision*, 20, 113–133.

Guzman, A. (1968) Decomposition of a visual scene into three-dimensional bodies. *Proceedings of AFIPS Conference*, 33, 291–304. Washington, DC: Thompson.

Hamlyn, D. W. (1961) *Sensation and perception*. New York: Routledge & Kegan Paul.

Haralick, R. M. & Shapiro, L. G. (1993) *Computer and robot vision*. New York: Addison-Wesley.

Hartley, R. & Zisserman, A. (2003) *Multiple view geometry in computer vision*. Cambridge: Cambridge University Press.

Hartline, H. K. & Ratliff, F. (1957) Inhibitory interaction of receptor units in the eye of limulus. *Journal of General Physiology*, 40, 357–376.

Hatfield, G. & Epstein, W. (1985) The status of the minimum principle in the theoretical analysis of visual perception. *Psychological Bulletin*, 97, 155–186.

Hay, C. J. (1966) Optical motions and space perception—An extension of Gibson's analysis. *Psychological Review*, 73, 550–565.

Hayward, W. G. & Tarr, M. J. (1997) Testing conditions for viewpoint invariance in object recognition. *Journal of Experimental Psychology: Human Perception and Performance*, 23, 1511–1521.

Hebb, D. O. (1949) *The organization of behavior*. New York: Wiley.

Helm, P. A. van der (2000) Simplicity versus likelihood in visual perception: From surprisals to precisals. *Psychological Bulletin*, 126, 770–800.

Helmholtz, H. von (1867/2000) *Treatise on physiological optics*. (Translated from German, J. P. C. Southall.) Bristol: Thoemmes.

Heidbreder, E. (1933) *Seven psychologies*. New York: Appleton.

Hick, W. E. (1952) On the rate of gain of information. *Quarterly Journal of Experimental Psychology*, 4, 11–26.

Hilbert, D. & Cohn-Vossen, S. (1952) *Geometry and the imagination*. New York: Chelsea Publishing Company.

Hildreth, E. C. (1984) The computation of the velocity field. *Proceedings of the Royal Society of London*, B221, 189–220.

Hillis, J. M., Watt, S. J., Landy, M. S. & Banks, M. S. (2004) Slant from texture and disparity cues: Optimal cue combination. *Journal of Vision*, 4, 1–24.

Hobbes, T. (1651) *Leviathan*. London.

Hochberg, J. (1972) Perception. In: Kling, J. W. & Riggs, L. A. (Eds.) *Woodworth and Schlosberg's experimental psychology* (pp. 395–550). New York: Holt, Rinehart & Winston.

Hochberg, J. (1978) *Perception*. Englewood Cliffs, NJ: Prentice-Hall.

Hochberg, J. & Brooks, V. (1960) The psychophysics of form: Reversible-perspective drawings of spatial objects. *American Journal of Psychology*, 73, 337–354.

Hochberg, J. & Brooks, V. (1962) Pictorial recognition as an unlearned ability: A study of one child's performance. *American Journal of Psychology*, 75, 624–628.

Hochberg, J. & McAlister, E. (1953) A quantitative approach to figural "goodness." *Journal of Experimental Psychology*, 46, 361–364.

Hoffman, D. D. & Richards, W. A. (1984) Parts of recognition. *Cognition*, 18, 65–96.

Holway, A. H. & Boring, E. G. (1941) Determinants of apparent visual size with distance variant. *American Journal of Psychology*, 54, 21–37.

Horn, B. K. P. (1975) Obtaining shape from shading information. In: Winston, P. H. (Ed.) *Psychology of computer vision* (pp. 115–155). New York: McGraw-Hill.

Horn, B. K. P. (1977) Understanding image intensities. *Artificial Intelligence*, 8, 201–231.

Howard, I. P. (1996) Alhazen's neglected discoveries of visual phenomena. *Perception*, 25, 1203–1217.

Howard, I. P. & Rogers, B. J. (1995) *Binocular vision and stereopsis*. New York: Oxford University Press.

Hubel, D. & Wiesel, T. (1962) Receptive fields, binocular interaction, and functional architecture in the cat's visual cortex. *Journal of Physiology*, 160, 106–154.

Huffman, D. A. (1971) Impossible objects as nonsense sentences. In: Meltzer, B. & Michie, D. (Eds.) *Machine intelligence* (Vol. 6, pp. 295–323). Edinburgh: Edinburgh University Press.

Hull, C. L. (1930) Knowledge and purpose as habit mechanisms. *Psychological Review*, 37, 511–525.

Hull, C. L. (1937) Mind, mechanism, and adaptive behavior. *Psychological Review*, 44, 1–32.

Hume, D. (1739/1978) *A treatise of human nature.* Oxford: Oxford University Press.

Hummel, J., Biederman, I., Gerhardstein, P. & Hilton, H. (1988) From edges to geons: A connectionist approach. *Proceedings, Connectionist Summer School*, pp. 462–471, Carnegie Mellon University.

Ikeuchi, K. & Horn, B. K. P. (1981) Numerical shape from shading and occluding boundaries. *Artificial Intelligence*, 17, 141–184.

Ikeuchi, K. & Kanade, K. (1988) Automatic generation of object recognition programs. *Proceedings of the IEEE*, 76, 1016–1035.

Ioffe, S. & Forsyth, D. A. (2001) Probabilistic methods for finding people. *International Journal of Computer Vision*, 43, 45–68.

Ittelson, W. H. (1968) *The Ames demonstrations in perception.* New York: Hafner.

Jacobs, D. (2000) What makes viewpoint invariant properties perceptually salient?: A computational perspective. In: Boyer, K. L. & Sarkar, S. (Eds.) *Perceptual organization for artificial vision systems*, pp. 121–138. Boston: Kluwer.

Jacot-Descombes, A. & Pun, T. (1992) A probabilistic approach to 3-D inference of geons from a 2-D view. *Proceedings, SPIE Applications of Artificial Intelligence X: Machine Vision and Robotics*, pp. 579–588, Orlando, FL.

James, W. (1890/1950) *The principles of psychology.* New York: Dover.

Jeffress, L. A. (1951) *Cerebral mechanisms in behavior: The Hixon symposium.* New York: Hafner.

Johnston, E. P. (1991) Systematic distortions of shape from stereopsis. *Vision Research*, 31, 1351–1360.

Jolion, J. M. & Kropatsch, W. G. (1998) *Graph based representations in pattern recognition.* Wien: Springer-Verlag.

Jolion, J. M. & Rosenfeld, A. (1994) *A pyramidal framework for early vision.* Boston: Kluwer.

Julesz, B. (1960) Binocular depth perception of computer-generated patterns. *Bell System Technical Journal*, 39, 1125–1162.

Julesz, B. (1971) *Foundations of cyclopean perception*. Chicago: University of Chicago Press.

Kaiser, P. K. (1967) Perceived shape and its dependency on perceived slant. *Journal of Experimental Psychology*, 75, 345–353.

Kanade, T. (1981) Recovery of the three-dimensional shape of an object from a single view. *Artificial Intelligence*, 17, 409–460.

Kanade, T. & Kender, J. R. (1983) Mapping image properties into shape constraints: Skewed symmetry, affine-transformable patterns, and the shape-from-texture paradigm. In: Beck, J., Hope, B. & Rosenfeld, A. (Eds.) *Human and machine vision* (pp. 237–257). New York: Academic Press.

Kanatani, K. (1988) Constraints on length and angle. *Computer Vision, Graphics, and Image Processing*, 41, 28–42.

Kanizsa, G. (1979) *Organization in vision*. New York: Praeger.

Kemp, M. (1990) *The science of art*. New Haven: Yale University Press.

Kepler, J. (1604/1966) Ad Vitellionem paralipomena. In: Herrnstein, R. J. & Boring, E. G. (Eds.) *A source book in the history of psychology* (pp. 91–97). Cambridge: Harvard University Press.

Kersten, D. (1990) Statistical limits to image understanding. In: Blakemore, C. (Ed.) *Vision coding and efficiency* (pp. 32–44). Cambridge: Cambridge University Press.

Kersten, D., Mamassian, P. & Yuille, A. (2004) Object perception as Bayesian inference. *Annual Review of Psychology*, 55, 271–304.

Kilpatrick, F. P. (1961) *Explorations in transactional psychology*. New York: New York University Press.

Kim, Z. W. & Nevatia, R. (1999) Uncertain reasoning and learning for feature grouping. *Computer Vision & Image Understanding*, 76, 278–288.

Klein, F. (1939) *Elementary mathematics from an advanced standpoint: Geometry*. New York: Dover.

Knill, D. C. (1992) Perception of surface contours and surface shape: From computation to psychophysics. *Journal of the Optical Society of America*, A9, 1449–1464.

Knill, D. C. (2001) Contour into texture: information content of surface contours and texture flow. *Journal of the Optical Society of America*, A18, 12–35.

Knill, D. C. & Richards, W. (1996) *Perception as Bayesian inference*. Cambridge: Cambridge University Press.

Knill, D. C. & Saunders, J. A. (2003) Do humans optimally integrate stereo and texture information for judgments of surface slant? *Vision Research*, 43, 2539–2558.

Koenderink, J. J. (1995) *Solid shape*. Cambridge: MIT Press.

Koenderink, J. J. & van Doorn, A. J. (1979) The internal representation of solid shape with respect to vision. *Biological Cybernetics*, 32, 211–216.

Koenderink, J. J. & van Doorn, A. J. (1991) Affine structure from motion. *Journal of the Optical Society of America*, 8, 377–385.

Koenderink, J. J. & van Doorn, A. J. (1995) Relief: Pictorial and otherwise. *Image and Vision Computing*, 13, 321–334.

Koenderink, J. J., van Doorn, A. J. & Kappers, A. M. L. (1992) Surface perception in pictures. *Perception & Psychophysics*, 52, 487–496.

Koenderink, J. J., van Doorn, A. J. & Kappers, A. M. L. (1994) On so-called paradoxical monocular stereoscopy. *Perception*, 23, 583–594.

Koenderink, J. J., van Doorn, A. J. & Kappers, A. M. L. (1995) Depth relief. *Perception*, 24, 115–126.

Koenderink, J. J., van Doorn, A. J. & Kappers, A. M. L. (1996) Pictorial surface attitude and local depth comparisons. *Perception & Psychophysics*, 58, 163–173.

Koenderink, J. J., van Doorn, A. J., Kappers, A. M. L. & Todd, J. T. (1997) The visual contour in depth. *Perception & Psychophysics*, 59, 828–838.

Koffka, K. (1935) *Principles of Gestalt psychology*. New York: Harcourt, Brace.

Kohler, I. (1962) Experiments with goggles. *Scientific American*, 206(5), 62–86.

Köhler, W. (1920/1938) *Physical Gestalten*. In: Ellis, W. D. (Ed.) *A source book of Gestalt psychology* (pp. 17–54). New York: Routledge & Kegan Paul.

Köhler, W. & Wallach, H. (1944) Figural after-effects: An investigation of visual processes. *Proceedings of the American Philosophical Society*, 88, 269–357.

Kontsevich, L. L. (2002) Symmetry as a depth cue. In: Tyler, C. W. (Ed.) *Human symmetry perception and its computational analysis* (pp. 331–347). Mahwah, NJ: Lawrence Erlbaum.

Kopfermann, H. (1930) Psychologische Untersuchungen über die Wirkung zweidimensionaler Darstellungen körperlicher Gebilde. *Psychologische Forschung*, 13, 293–364.

Kriegman, D. & Ponce, J. (1990) Computing exact aspect graphs of curved objects: Solids of revolution. *International Journal of Computer Vision*, 5, 119–135.

Kuffler, S. W. (1953) Discharge patterns and functional organization of mammalian retina. *Journal of Neurophysiology*, 16, 37–68.

Lamdan, Y., Schwartz, J. T. & Wolfson, H. J. (1988) Object recognition by affine invariant matching. *Proceedings of the IEEE Conference on Computer Vision & Pattern Recognition*, pp. 335–344.

Lanczos, C. (1970) *The variational principles of mechanics*. New York: Dover.

Landy, M. S., Maloney, L. T., Johnston, E. B. & Young, M. (1995) Measurement and modeling of depth cue combination: In defense of weak fusion. *Vision Research, 35*, 389–412.

Leclerc, Y. G. (1989) Constructing simple stable descriptions for image partitioning. *International Journal of Computer Vision, 3*, 73–102.

Leclerc, Y. G. & Fischler, M. A. (1992) An optimization-based approach to the interpretation of single line drawings as 3D wire frames. *International Journal of Computer Vision, 9*, 113–136.

Leeuwenberg, E. L. J. (1971) A perceptual coding language for visual and auditory patterns. *Amercian Journal of Psychology, 84*, 307–349.

Leibowitz, H. W. & Bourne, L. E. (1956) Time and intensity as determiners of perceived shape. *Journal of Experimental Psychology, 51*, 277–281.

Leibowitz, H. W., Wilcox, S. B. & Post, R. B. (1978) The effect of refractive error on size constancy and shape constancy. *Perception, 7*, 557–562.

Lettvin, J. Y., Maturana, H. R., McCulloch, W. S. & Pitts, W. H. (1951) What the frog's eye tells the frog's brain. *Proceedings of the Institute of Radio Engineers, 47*, 1940–1959.

Levine, M. W. (2000) *Fundamentals of sensation and perception*. New York: Oxford University Press.

Li, M. & Vitanyi, P. (1997) *An introduction to Kolmogorov complexity and its applications*. New York: Springer.

Li, Y. & Pizlo, Z. (2005) Monocular and binocular perception of 3D shape: The role of *a priori* constraints. *Annual Meeting of the Vision Sciences Society*.

Li, Y. & Pizlo, Z. (2006) Is viewer-centered representation necessary for 3D shape perception? *Annual Meeting of the Vision Sciences Society*.

Li, Y. & Pizlo, Z. (2007) Reconstruction of shapes of 3D symmetric objects by using planarity and compactness constraints. *Proceedings of IS&T/SPIE Electronic Imaging Symposium, Conference on Vision Geometry*, vol. 6499.

Linden, D. E. J., Kallenbach, U., Heinecke, A., Singer, W. & Goebel, R. (1999) The myth of upright vision. A psychophysical and functional imaging study of adaptation to inverting spectacles. *Perception, 28*, 469–481.

Liu, Z. & Kersten, D. (1998) 2D observers for human 3D object recognition? *Vision Research, 38*, 2507–2519.

Liu, Z., Knill, D. C. & Kersten, D. (1995) Object classification for human and ideal observers. *Vision Research, 35*, 549–568.

Locke, J. (1690/1975) *An essay concerning human understanding*. Oxford: Clarendon.

Longuet-Higgins, H. C. (1981) A computer algorithm for reconstructing a scene from two projections. *Nature*, 293, 133–135.

Lotka, A. J. (1925/1956) *Elements of mathematical biology*. New York: Dover.

Lotze, H. (1852/1886) *Outlines of psychology*. Boston: Ginn.

Lowe, D. G. (1985) *Perceptual organization and visual recognition*. Boston: Kluwer.

Luce, R. D. (2003) Whatever happened to information theory in psychology? *Review of General Psychology*, 7, 183–188.

Luneburg, R. K. (1947) *Mathematical analysis of binocular vision*. Princeton: Princeton University Press.

Mach, E. (1906/1959) *The analysis of sensations*. New York: Dover.

Mackworth, A. K. (1973) Interpreting pictures of polyhedral scenes. *Artificial Intelligence*, 4, 121–137.

Macmillan, N. A. & Creelman, C. D. (2005) *Detection theory: A user's guide*. Mahwah, NJ: Lawrence Erlbaum.

Malik, J. & Maydan, D. (1989) Recovering three-dimensional shape from a single image of curved objects. *IEEE Transactions on Pattern Analysis and Machine Intelligence*, 11, 555–566.

Mamassian, P. & Landy, M. S. (1998) Observer biases in the 3D interpretation of line drawings. *Vision Research*, 38, 2817–2832.

Marill, T. (1991) Emulating the human interpretation of line drawings as three-dimensional objects. *International Journal of Computer Vision*, 6, 147–161.

Marr, D. (1977) Analysis of occluding contour. *Proceedings of the Royal Society of London*, B197, 441–475.

Marr, D. (1982) *Vision*. New York: W.H. Freeman.

Marr, D. & Nishihara, H. K. (1978) Representation and recognition of the spatial organization of three-dimensional shapes. *Proceedings of the Royal Society of London*, B200, 269–294.

Mayr, O. (1970) *The origins of feedback control*. Cambridge: MIT Press.

McCulloch, W. S. & Pitts, W. (1943) A logical calculus of the ideas immanent in nervous activity. *Bulletin of Mathematical Biophysics*, 5, 115–133.

McKee, S. P., Levi, D. M. & Bowne, S. F. (1990) The imprecision of stereopsis. *Vision Research*, 30, 1763–1779.

Meneghini, K. A. & Leibowitz, H. W. (1967) Effect of stimulus distance and age on shape constancy. *Journal of Experimental Psychology*, 74, 241–248.

Miller, G. A. (1951) *Language and communication*. New York: McGraw-Hill.

Miller, G. A. (1956) The magical number seven, plus or minus two: Some limits on our capacity for processing information. *Psychological Review*, 63, 81–97.

Miller, G. A., Galanter, E. & Pribram, K. H. (1960) *Plans and the structure of behavior*. New York: Holt.

Miller, G. A. & Selfridge, J. A. (1950) Verbal context and the recall of meaningful material. *American Journal of Psychology*, 63, 176–185.

Miller, J. & Festinger, L. (1977) Impact of oculomotor retraining on the visual perception of curvature. *Journal of Experimental Psychology: Human Perception and Performance*, 3, 187–200.

Minsky, M. (1968) *Semantic information processing*. Cambridge: MIT Press.

Minsky, M. (1975) A framework for representing knowledge. In: Winston, P. H. (Ed.) *The psychology of computer vision* (pp. 211–277). New York: McGraw-Hill.

Minsky, M. & Pappert, S. (1969) *Perceptrons: An introduction to computational geometry*. Cambridge: MIT Press.

Molyneux, W. (1692) *A treatise of dioptricks*. London.

Mundy, J. L. & Zisserman, A. (1992) *Geometric invariance in computer vision*. Cambridge: MIT Press.

Mundy, J. L., Zisserman, A. & Forsyth, D. (1993) *Applications of invariance in computer vision*. New York: Springer-Verlag.

Munck-Fairwood, R. (1991) Recognition of generic components using logic-program relations of image contours. *Image and Vision Computing*, 9, 113–122.

Munck-Fairwood, R. & Barreau, G. (1991) A belief network for the recognition of 3D geometric primitives. *Proceedings, 6th International Conference on Image Analysis and Processing*, Como, Italy.

Münsterberg, H. (1914) *Psychology: General and applied*. New York: Appleton.

Nagel, E. (1961) *The structure of science. Problems in the logic of scientific explanation*. New York: Harcourt, Brace & World.

Nefs, H. T., Koenderink, J. J. & Kappers, A. M. L. (2005) The influence of illumination direction on the pictorial reliefs of Lambertian surfaces. *Perception*, 34, 275–287.

Neisser, U. (1967) *Cognitive psychology*. New York: Appleton.

Neuman, J. von (1951) The general and logical theory of automata. In: Jeffress, L. A. (Ed.) *Cerebral mechanisms in behavior* (pp. 1–31). New York: Hafner.

Nevatia, R. (2000) Perceptual organization for generic object description. In: Boyer, K. L. & Sarkar, S. (Eds.) *Perceptual organization for artificial vision systems* (pp. 173–189). Boston: Kluwer.

Norman, J. F., Todd, J. T., Perotti, V. J. & Tittle, J. S. (1996) The visual perception of three-dimensional length. *Journal of Experimental Psychology: Human Perception and Performance*, 22, 173–186.

Noton, D. & Stark, L. (1971) Scanpaths in eye movements during pattern perception. *Science*, 171, 308–311.

Palmer, S. E. (1985) The role of symmetry in shape perception. *Acta Psychologica*, 59, 67–90.

Palmer, S. E. (1999) *Vision science*. Cambridge: MIT Press.

Palmer, S. E., Rosch, E. & Chase, P. (1981) Canonical perspective and the perception of objects. In: Long, J. & Baddeley, A. (Eds.) *Attention and Performance* (Vol. 9, pp. 135–151). Hillsdale, NJ: Lawrence Erlbaum.

Papathomas, T. V. (2002) Experiments on the role of pictorial cues in Hughes' reversperspectives. *Perception*, 31, 521–530.

Pastore, N. (1971) *Selective history of theories of visual perception: 1650–1950*. New York: Oxford University Press.

Pelillo, M., Siddiqi, K. & Zucker, S. W. (1999) Matching hierarchical structures using association graphs. *IEEE Transactions on Pattern Analysis and Machine Intelligence*, 21, 1105–1120.

Penrose, L. S. & Penrose, R. (1958) Impossible objects: A special type of visual illusion. *British Journal of Psychology*, 49, 31–33.

Pentland, A. P. (1986) Perceptual organization and the representation of natural form. *Artificial Intelligence*, 28, 293–331.

Perkins, D. N. (1972) Visual discrimination between rectangular and nonrectangular parallelopipeds. *Perception & Psychophysics*, 12, 396–400.

Perkins, D. N. (1976) How good a bet is good form? *Perception*, 5, 393–406.

Perkins, D. N. & Cooper, R. G. (1980) How the eye makes up what the light leaves out. In: Hagen, M. A. (Ed.) *The perception of pictures* (Vol. 2, pp. 95–130). New York: Academic Press.

Perrone, J. A. (1980) Slant underestimation: A model based on the size of the viewing aperture. *Perception*, 9, 285–302.

Perrone, J. A. (1982) Visual slant underestimation: A general model. *Perception*, 11, 641–654.

Pitt, M. A., Myung, J. & Zhang, S. (2002) Toward a method of selecting among computational models of cognition. *Psychological Review*, 109, 472–491.

Pitts, W. & McCulloch, W. S. (1947) How we know universals: The perception of auditory and visual forms. *Bulletin of Mathematical Biophysics*, 9, 127–147.

Pizlo, Z. (1994) A theory of shape constancy based on perspective invariants. *Vision Research*, 34, 1637–1658.

Pizlo, Z. (2001) Perception viewed as an inverse problem. *Vision Research*, 41, 3145–3161.

Pizlo, Z., Li, Y. & Chan, M. W. (2005) Regularization model of human binocular vision. *Proceedings of IS&T/SPIE Conference on Computational Imaging*, 5674, 229–240.

Pizlo, Z., Li, Y. & Francis, G. (2005) A new look at binocular stereopsis. *Vision Research*, 45, 2244–2255.

Pizlo, Z., Li, Y. & Steinman, R. M. (2006) A new paradigm for 3D shape perception. *European Conference on Visual Perception*. St. Petersburg, Russia.

Pizlo, Z. & Loubier, K. (2000) Recognition of a solid shape from its single perspective image obtained by a calibrated camera. *Pattern Recognition*, 33, 1675–1681.

Pizlo, Z. & Rosenfeld, A. (1990) Recognition of planar shapes from perspective images using contour-based invariants. Center for Automation Research, CAR-TR-528. University of Maryland, College Park, MD.

Pizlo, Z. & Rosenfeld, A. (1992) Recognition of planar shapes from perspective images using contour-based invariants. *Computer Vision, Graphics, and Image Processing: Image Understanding*, 56, 330–350.

Pizlo, Z., Rosenfeld, A. & Weiss, I. (1995) Interdisciplinary study of visual invariants. In: Dori, D. & Bruckstein, A. (Eds.) *Shape, structure and pattern recognition* (pp. 118–127). London: World Scientific.

Pizlo, Z., Rosenfeld, A. & Weiss, I. (1997a) The geometry of visual space: About the incompatibility between science and mathematics. Dialogue. *Computer Vision & Image Understanding*, 65, 425–433.

Pizlo, Z., Rosenfeld, A. & Weiss, I. (1997b) Visual space: Mathematics, engineering, and science. Response. *Computer Vision & Image Understanding*, 65, 450–454.

Pizlo, Z. & Salach-Golyska, M. (1995) 3D shape perception. *Perception & Psychophysics*, 57, 692–714.

Pizlo, Z. & Scheessele, M. R. (1998) Perception of 3D scenes from pictures. *IS&T/SPIE Proceedings of Electronic Imaging Conference*, 3299, 410–423.

Pizlo, Z. & Stevenson, A. K. (1999) Shape constancy from novel views. *Perception & Psychophysics*, 61, 1299–1307.

Plantinga, H. & Dyer, C. (1990) Visibility, occlusion, and the aspect graph. *International Journal of Computer Vision*, 5, 137–160.

Poggio, T. & Edelman, S. (1990) A network that learns to recognize three-dimensional objects. *Nature*, 343, 263–266.

Poggio, T., Torre, V. & Koch, C. (1985) Computational vision and regularization theory. *Nature*, 317, 314–319.

Polya, G. & Szego, G. (1951) *Isoperimetric inequalities in mathematical physics*. Princeton: Princeton University Press.

Polyak, S. (1957) *The vertebrate visual system*. Chicago: University of Chicago Press.

Popper, K. R. (1979) *Objective knowledge*. Oxford: Oxford University Press.

Raja, N. & Jain, A. (1992) Recognizing geons from superquadrics fitted to range data. *Image and Vision Computing*, 10, 179–190.

Raja, N. & Jain, A. (1994) Obtaining generic parts from range images using a multiview representation. *CVGIP: Image Understanding*, 60, 44–64.

Regan, D. (2000) *Human perception of objects*. Sunderland, MA: Sinauer.

Richards, W. (1990) In: Vaina, L. M. (Ed.) *From the retina to the neocortex: Selected papers of David Marr*. Boston: Springer Verleg.

Roberts, L. G. (1965) Machine perception of three-dimensional solids. In: Tippett, J. T. et al. (Eds.) *Optical and electro-optical information processing* (pp. 159–197). Cambridge: MIT Press.

Rock, I. (1973) *Orientation and form*. New York: Academic Press.

Rock, I. (1977) In defense of unconscious inference. In: Epstein, W. (Ed.) Stability and constancy in visual perception (pp. 321–373). New York: Wiley.

Rock, I. (1983) *The logic of perception*. Cambridge: MIT Press.

Rock, I. & DiVita, J. (1987) A case of viewer-centered object perception. *Cognitive Psychology*, 19, 280–293.

Rock, I., DiVita, J. & Barbeito, R. (1981) The effect on form perception of change of orientation in the third dimension. *Journal of Experimental Psychology: Human Perception and Performance*, 7, 719–732.

Rock, I., Wheeler, D. & Tudor, L. (1989) Can we imagine how objects look from other viewpoints? *Cognitive Psychology*, 21, 185–210.

Rosenblatt, F. (1962) *Principles of neurodynamics*. Washington, DC: Spartan Books.

Rosenblueth, A., Wiener, N. & Bigelow, J. (1943) Behavior, purpose and teleology. *Philosophy of Science*, 10, 18–24.

Rothwell, C. A. (1995) *Object recognition through invariant indexing*. Oxford: Oxford University Press.

Rothwell, C. A., Forsyth, D. A., Zisserman, A. & Mundy, J. L. (1993) Extracting projective structure from single perspective views of 3D point sets. *Proceedings of the IEEE International Conference on Computer Vision*, pp. 573–582.

Rumelhart, D. E. & McClelland, J. L. (1986) *Parallel distributed processing*. Cambridge: MIT Press.

Sabra, A. I. (1989) *The optics of Ibn Al-Haytham*. London: Warburg Institute.

Sabra, A. I. (1994) *Optics, astronomy and logic: Studies in Arabic science and philosophy*. Aldershot: Variorum.

Sallam, M. & Bowyer, K. (1991) Generalizing the aspect graph concept to include articulated assemblies. *Pattern Recognition Letters*, 12, 171–176.

Saunders, J. A. & Knill, D. C. (2001) Perception of 3D surface orientation from skew symmetry. *Vision Research*, 41, 3163–3183.

Scarfe, P. & Hibbard, P. B. (2006) Disparity-defined objects moving in depth do not elicit three-dimensional shape constancy. *Vision Research*, 46, 1599–1610.

Schiffman, H. R. (2001) *Sensation and perception*. New York: Wiley.

Schrater, P. R. & Kersten, D. (2000) How optimal depth cue integration depends on the task. *International Journal of Computer Vision*, 40, 73–91.

Schriever, W. (1925) Experimentelle Studien über stereoskopisches Schen. *Zeitschrift für Psychologie*, 96, 113–170.

Sebastian, T. B., Klein, P. N. & Kimia, B. B. (2004) Recognition of shapes by editing their shock graphs. *IEEE Transactions on Pattern Analysis and Machine Intelligence*, 26, 505–571.

Selfridge, O. G. & Neisser, U. (1960) Pattern recognition by machine. *Scientific American*, 203(8), 60–68.

Senden, M. von (1932/1960) *Space and sight*. London: Methuen.

Shannon, C. E. (1948) A mathematical theory of communication. *The Bell System Technical Journal*, 27, 379–423, 623–656.

Shepard, R. N. (1981) Psychophysical complementarity. In: Kubovy, M. & Pomerantz, J. R. (Eds.) *Perceptual organization* (pp. 279–341). Hillsdale, NJ: Lawrence Erlbaum.

Shepard, R. N. & Cooper, L. A. (1982) *Mental images and their transformations*. Cambridge: MIT Press.

Shepard, R. N. & Metzler, J. (1971) Mental rotation of three-dimensional objects. *Science*, 171, 701–703.

Shimshoni, I. & Ponce, J. (1993) Finite resolution aspect graphs of polyhedral objects. *Proceedings, IEEE Workshop on Qualitative Vision*, pp. 140–150. New York, NY.

Siddiqi, K., Shokoufandeh, A., Dickinson, S. J. & Zucker, S. W. (1999) Shock graphs and shape matching. *International Journal of Computer Vision*, 35, 13–32.

Sinha P. (1995) Perceiving and recognizing three-dimensional forms. Doctoral dissertation. Massachusetts Institute of Technology. Dept. of Electrical Engineering and Computer Science.

Sinha, P. & Adelson, E. H. (1992) Recovery of 3-D shape from 2-D wireframe drawings. *Investigative Ophthalmology & Visual Science*, 33 (Suppl.), 825.

Slater A. & Morison V. (1985) Shape constancy and slant perception at birth. *Perception*, 14, 337–344.

Stankiewicz, B. J. (2002) Empirical evidence for independent dimensions in the visual representation of three-dimensional shape. *Journal of Experimental Psychology: Human Perception and Performance*, 28, 913–932.

Stavrianos, B. K. (1945) The relation of shape perception to explicit judgments of inclination. *Archives of Psychology*, 296, 1–94.

Steinman, R. M., Pizlo, Z. & Pizlo, F. J. (2000) Phi is not beta, and why Wertheimer's discovery launched the Gestalt revolution. *Vision Research*, 40, 2237–2264.

Stevens, K. A. (1981) The visual interpretation of surface contours. *Artificial Intelligence*, 17, 47–73.

Stevens, K. A. (1983) Surface tilt (the direction of slant): A neglected psychophysical variable. *Perception and Psychophysics*, 33, 241–250.

Stevens, K. (1986) Inferring shape from contours across surfaces. In: Pentland, A. P. (Ed.) *From pixels to predicates* (pp. 93–110). Norwood, NJ: Ablex Publishing Corporation.

Stevens, K. A. & Brookes, A. (1988) Integrating stereopsis with monocular interpretations of planar surfaces. *Vision Research*, 28, 371–386.

Stevens, K. A. Lees, M. & Brookes, A. (1991) Combining binocular and monocular curvature features. *Perception*, 20, 425–440.

Stewman, J. & Bowyer, K. (1990) Direct construction of the perspective projection aspect graph of convex polyhedra. *Computer Vision, Graphics, and Image Processing*, 51, 20–37.

Stratton, G. M. (1896) Some preliminary experiments on vision without inversion of the retinal image. *Psychological Review*, 3, 611–617.

Sugihara, K. (1986) *Machine interpretation of line drawings*. Cambridge: MIT Press.

Talbot, S. A. & Marshall, W. H. (1941) Physiological studies on neural mechanisms of visual localization and discrimination. *American Journal of Ophthalmology*, 24, 1255–1264.

Tarr, M. J., Bülthoff, H. H., Zabinski, M. & Blanz, V. (1997) To what extent do unique parts influence recognition across changes in viewpoint? *Psychological Science*, 8, 282–289.

Tarr, M. J. & Pinker, S. (1991) Orientation-dependent mechanisms in shape recognition. *Psychological Science*, 2, 207–209.

Tarr, M. J., Williams, P., Hayward, W. G. & Gauthier, I. (1998) Three-dimensional object recognition is viewpoint dependent. *Nature Neuroscience*, 1, 275–277.

Thompson, D'Arcy W. (1942/1992) *On growth and form*. New York: Dover.

Thouless, R. H. (1931a) Phenomenal regression to the real object. I. *British Journal of Psychology*, 21, 339–359.

Thouless, R. H. (1931b) Phenomenal regression to the real object. II. *British Journal of Psychology*, 22, 1–30.

Thouless, R. H. (1934) The general principle underlying effects attributed to the so-called phenomenal constancy tendency. *Psychologische Forschung*, 19, 300–310.

Tikhonov, A. N. & Arsenin, V. Y. (1977) *Solutions of ill-posed problems*. New York: Wiley.

Tittle, J. S., Todd, J. T., Perotti, V. J. & Norman, J. F. (1995) Systematic distortion of perceived three-dimensional structure from motion and stereopsis. *Journal of Experimental Psychology: Human Perception and Performance*, 21, 663–678.

Tjan, B. S. & Legge, G. E. (1998) The viewpoint complexity of an object-recognition task. *Vision Research*, 38, 2335–2350.

Todd, J. T., Koenderink, J. J., van Doorn, A. J. & Kappers, A. M. L. (1996) Effects of changing viewing conditions on the perceived structure of smoothly curved surfaces. *Journal of Experimental Psychology: Human Perception and Performance*, 22, 695–706.

Todd, J. T. & Norman, J. F. (2003) The visual perception of 3D shape from multiple cues: Are observers capable of perceiving metric structure? *Perception & Psychophysics*, 65, 31–47.

Tolman, E. C. (1932) *Purposive behavior in animals and men*. New York: Century.

Treisman, A. & Gelade, G. (1980) A feature integration theory of attention. *Cognitive Psychology*, 12, 97–136.

Tsai, R. Y. & Huang, T. S. (1984) Uniqueness and estimation of 3D motion parameters of rigid objects with curved surfaces. *IEEE Transactions on Pattern Analysis and Machine Intelligence*, 6, 13–27.

Turing, A. M. (1936) On computable numbers with an application to the Entscheidungsproblem. *Proceedings of the London Mathematical Society*, Series 2, 42, 230–265.

Ullman, S. (1979) *The interpretation of visual motion*. Cambridge: MIT Press.

Ullman, S. (1980) Against direct perception. *Behavioral and Brain Sciences*, 3, 373–415.

Ulupinar, F. & Nevatia, R. (1995) Shape from contour: Straight homogeneous generalized cylinders and constant cross section generalized cylinders. *IEEE Transactions on Pattern Analysis and Machine Intelligence*, 17, 120–135.

Vetter, T. & Poggio, T. (2002) Symmetric 3D objects are an easy case for 2D object recognition. In: Tyler, C. W. (Ed.) *Human symmetry perception and its computational analysis* (pp. 349–359). Mahwah, NJ: Lawrence Erlbaum.

Wagemans, J., van Gool, L. & Lamote, C. (1996) The visual system's measurement of invariants need not itself be invariant. *Psychological Science*, 7, 232–236.

Wagemans, J., van Gool, L., Lamote, C. & Foster, D. H. (2000) Minimal information to determine affine shape equivalence. *Journal of Experimental Psychology: Human Perception and Performance*, 26, 443–468.

Wallach, H. (1976) *On perception*. New York: Quadrangle.

Wallach, H. & Moore, M. E. (1962) The role of slant in the perception of shape. *American Journal of Psychology*, 75, 289–293.

Wallach, H. & O'Connell, D. N. (1953) The kinetic depth effect. *Journal of Experimental Psychology*, 45, 205–217.

Wallach, H. O'Connell, D. N. & Neisser, U. (1953) The memory effect of visual perception of three-dimensional form. *Journal of Experimental Psychology*, 45, 360–368.

Walsh, V. & Kulikowski, J. (1998) *Perceptual constancy*. Cambridge: Cambridge University Press.

Waltz, D. (1972/1975) Understanding line drawings of scenes with shadows. In: Winston, P. H. *The psychology of computer vision*. (pp. 19–91). New York: McGraw-Hill.

Warren, H. C. (1916) A study of purpose. I. *The Journal of Philosophy, Psychology and Scientific Methods*, 13, 5–26.

Watt, R. J. (1987) Scanning from coarse to fine spatial scales in the human visual system after the onset of the stimulus. *Journal of the Optical Society of America*, A4, 2006–2021.

Weinshall, D. (1993) Model-based invariants for 3-D vision. *International Journal of Computer Vision*, 10, 27–42.

Weiss, I. (1988a) Projective invariants of shapes. *Proceedings of DARPA Image Understanding Workshop* (pp. 1125–1134). Cambridge, MA.

Weiss, I. (1988b) 3D shape representation by contours. *Computer Vision, Graphics, and Image Processing*, 41, 80–100.

Weiss, I. (1993) Geometric invariants and object recognition. *International Journal of Computer Vision*, 10, 207–231.

Wertheimer, M. (1912) Experimentelle Studien über das Sehen von Bewegung. *Zeitschrift für Psychologie*, 61, 161–265.

Wertheimer, M. (1923/1958) Principles of perceptual organization. In: Beardslee, D. C. & Wertheimer, M. (Eds.) *Readings in perception* (pp. 115–135). New York: D. van Nostrand.

Wiener, N. (1948) *Cybernetics*. Cambridge: MIT Press.

Witkin, A. P. (1981) Recovering surface shape and orientation from texture. *Artificial Intelligence*, 17, 17–45.

Witkin, A. P., Terzopulos, D. & Kaas, M. (1987) Signal matching through scale space. *International Journal of Computer Vision*, 1, 133–144.

Woodworth, R. S. (1938) *Experimental psychology*. New York: Holt.

Wu, K. & Levine, M. (1994) Recovering parametric geons from multiview range data. *Proceedings, IEEE Conference on Computer Vision and Pattern Recognition*, pp. 159–166, Seattle, WA.

Zerroug, M. & Nevatia, R. (1996) Three-dimensional descriptions based on the analysis of the invariant and quasi-invariant properties of some curved-axis generalized cylinders. *IEEE Transactions on Pattern Analysis and Machine Intelligence*, 18, 237–253.

Zerroug, M. & Nevatia, R. (1999) Part-based 3D descriptions of complex objects from a single image. *IEEE Transactions on Pattern Analysis and Machine Intelligence*, 21, 835–848.

Zuckermann, C. B. & Rock, I. A. (1957) A reappraisal of the role of past experience and innate organizing processes in visual perception. *Psychological Bulletin*, 54, 269–296.

Zusne, L. (1970) *Visual perception of form*. New York: Academic Press.

Index